Yoga

Sophy Hoare

Macdonald Guidelines

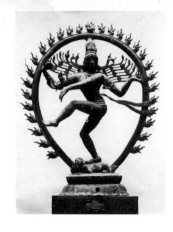
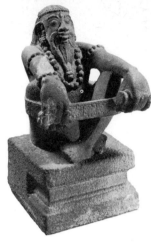

Editorial manager
Chester Fisher
Series editor
Jim Miles
Designer
Barry Kemp
Production
Philip Hughes
Picture research
Maggie Colbeck

Made and printed by
Waterlow (Dunstable) Ltd

ISBN 0 356 06012 8

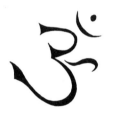

First published 1977
Macdonald Educational Ltd
Holywell House,
Worship Street,
London EC2A 2EN

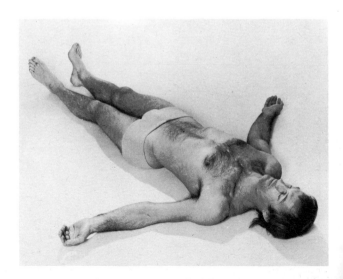

Contents

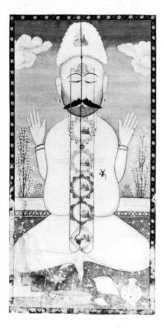

Information

4 What is yoga?
6 The origins of yoga
10 Yoga philosophy
14 Types of yoga
26 Yoga and science
28 Yoga today

Activities

32 Preparing for action
35 The postures
80 Pranayama—breathing
81 Meditation

Reference

84 Planning a programme
86 List of postures
88 Yoga for health
90 Courses and addresses
91 Glossary
94 Index

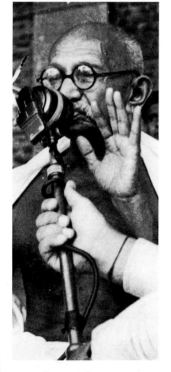

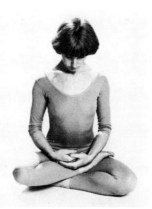

What is yoga?

Yoga is a very ancient practice which originated in India. It consists of physical and mental disciplines which make us healthy, alert and receptive, transforming our perception of the world and the way we live in it. Yoga has grown and been amended continuously through thousands of years to meet the changing conditions of mankind; but it has always been directed to allowing the individual to achieve his or her full potential as a human being, and then to stretch beyond into spiritual consciousness.

The word yoga comes from the same Sanskrit root as the word yoke. Hence it implies the harnessing of oneself to a discipline or a way of life. Yoga can be used at any level of living. It is often said that there are as many yogas as there are yogis, because the system can be infinitely adjusted by each person to suit themselves. There are many forms of yoga to cover the many areas of human activity, but they are all closely interrelated. In fact one of the chief purposes is to create a well-integrated person who can live with health and happiness among his fellow beings. One of the central ideas of yoga—because it is revealed through practising yoga—is the interdependence of all things, animate and inanimate, in the entire universe. Nothing can be taken in isolation. In the words of the poet John Donne, "No man is an island". This sense of the oneness of all things is often understood to be the "yoking" or "union" implied in the word yoga.

Although anyone of whatever religion or belief can be a yogi, the historical background of yoga is mainly in the Hindu tradition. Thus, when yogis have achieved the mystic experience known as "Samadhi" or superconsciousness, it has been interpreted in Hindu terms as contact with Brahman, the universal spirit.

Samadhi is an individual experience, but the descriptions of it correspond closely to the mystic experiences of religions in other cultures, which explains why yoga is often mistaken for a religion. Yoga is not a religion, for it does not demand adherence to any one dogma in the form of faith in a prophet or "divinely inspired" writings.

Yoga is a technique of personal development which existed long before any system of philosophy. To find out what yoga is, the simplest way is to practise it. In this way one can recognise the many faces of yoga as they are described in the Bhagavadgita, a great work on yoga from the sixth century BC, which are:

Yoga is equilibrium in success and failure.

Yoga is skilful living among activities.

Yoga is the supreme secret of life.

Yoga is the producer of the greatest happiness.

Yoga is effected by self-control.

Yoga is non-attachment.

Yoga is the destroyer of pain.

Yoga is serenity.

▶ This seventeenth century picture depicting Krishna in various guises shows him as a yogi in the bottom left corner, seated on the traditional yoga mat, a tiger skin.

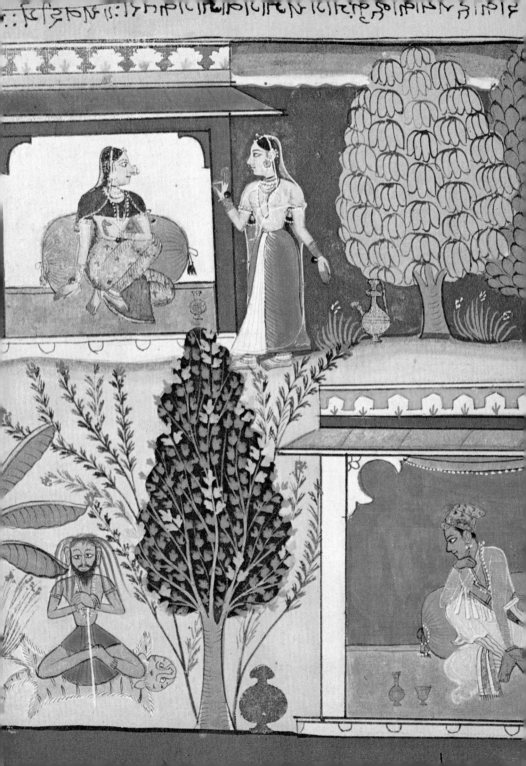

The origins of yoga

The history of yoga is not well charted. In India, where yoga originated, the study of history has never had the importance accorded to it in the West, for Indian thought has traditionally been more concerned with transcending time than recording it. Those historians who have delved into the background of yoga have found it hard if not impossible to establish facts such as the dates and authorship of works on the subject.

The earliest evidence of yoga is archaeological. Excavations begun in the twenties have revealed signs of an ancient civilization which flourished in India as early as 3000 BC and perhaps earlier. Among the finds are some stone seals showing godlike figures in yogic postures, one of which has been identified with the Hindu god Shiva, the mythological founder of yoga. Yoga techniques may have existed long before the arrival of the Aryan tribes whose domination shaped the development of Hinduism.

The earliest reference to yoga as a technical term occurs in the literature of the Vedas. This is a collection of hymns and philosophical poetry which was composed over the huge period of 2000 years and was transmitted orally long before it was written down. The Vedas reflect the evolution of early Indian religious thought, from a polytheistic nature worship in which ritual sacrifice played a central role, to a religion which recognized one absolute reality which was infinite and all-pervading. The supreme principle became not one all-

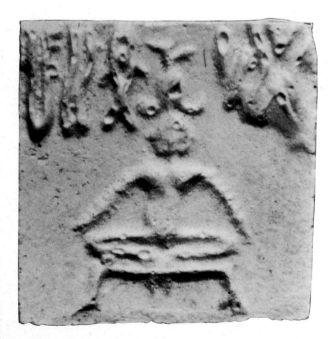

◀ One of the oldest known portrayals of a yogi. This figure on a stone seal dates from about 2500 BC and was found on the site of Mohenjo-Daro in the Indus Valley. An ancient civilization flourished there long before the north of India was invaded by the Aryan tribes. The seals carry a script which has not yet been deciphered.

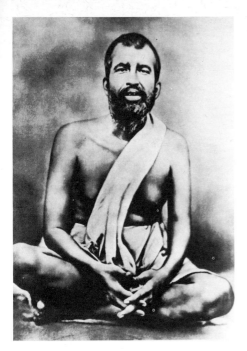

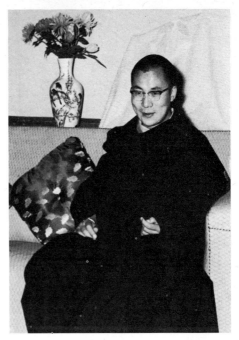

▲ Ramakrishna, a saint and yogi philospher who lived in the second half of the nineteenth century.

▲ The Dalai Lama, spiritual ruler of Tibet, a modern yogi revered by his followers as a divine incarnation.

powerful personal god, but an abstract concept of the Absolute. This is referred to in the earlier Vedas as That One (neuter Tad Ekam) and in the later part of the Vedas called the Upanishads, as Brahman.

The oneness of Brahman is the basis of the major school of Hindu philosophy, Vedanta, which is implied in many later works on yoga. It is expressed in the "great sentences" of the Upanishads, of which the best known is: "Tatt vam Asi", which means "That thou art"; in other words, everything is Brahman. This truth is realized through meditation, study and devotion — through the discipline of yoga. The Katha Upanishad says: "When the five senses and the mind are still, and reason itself rests in silence, then begins the Path Supreme. This calm steadiness of the senses is called Yoga".

Here is yoga described as a technique for achieving a higher state of awareness. In Hindu Veda means wisdom and the Vedas and Upanishads are considered in Hindu philosophy as divine revelations, truths revealed to the Rishis or ancient Seers. They are the roots of the philosophy within whose framework yoga developed, and they give us a glimpse of early yoga technique.

The Bhagavadgita

In the sixth century BC perhaps the greatest and best known work on yoga was written, the Bhagavadgita. This is one poem in a lengthy epic called the Mahabharata and it consists of a discourse by the god Krishna to the warrior Arjuna on the philosophy

7

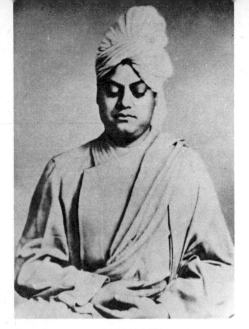

The Bhagavadgita was written around the time that the Buddha lived. At this time the main streams of philosophical thought in India were shaping into distinct systems. One of the "orthodox" Hindu systems was classical yoga, probably summarized in writing about the second century AD as the Yoga Sutras, ascribed to Patanjali. Two movements which grew into independent religions were Buddhism and Jainism. They separated from Hinduism because they evolved outside the latter's social and religious hierarchical structure. But they both

contemplative life. Though it is set in the Hindu philosophy, the way of life or yoga that it advocates could be followed, to their greater happiness, by people of any race or conviction.

Classical yoga

▲ Vivekenanda (1863-1902) was a distinguished scholar of philosophy who became a disciple of Ramakrishna. He renounced his wealth to become a Sannyasin, founded Ashrams (yoga schools) and spread Ramakrishna's teaching throughout the world. He was an enormously energetic man who probably more than any other person made the West familiar with Hinduism and yoga.

▶ Jain monks. Jainism is a religion about as old as Buddhism. Its central doctrine of Ahimsa, respect for all life, is taken to extremes. The monks wear masks to avoid breathing in and harming microscopic creatures.

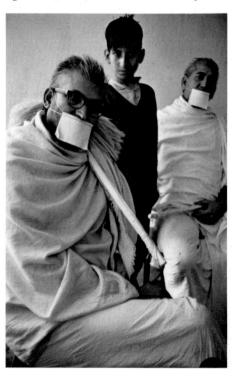

and practice of yoga. Krishna is symbolizing the cosmic aspect of Brahman. The Bhagavadgita describes several paths of yoga, the yoga of action, of devotion and of knowledge. It also describes the qualities of the ideal yogi, whatever his path. The work is characterized by its emphasis on achieving liberation through active life. It offers spiritual teaching to everyone, not only those who renounce the world for a incorporated yogic techniques, as did the many sects which developed within Hinduism during the first few centuries AD.

Yoga is not a religion

The tradition of yoga from very early times has been one of personal instruction from teacher to student. Because yoga is a technique of self-development which demands no dogmatic belief, only a faith in the individual's own potential, it has often been regarded with suspicion by the dogmatists of religion and society. There is a reference in the Vedas to a group of people called the Vratyas, who may have been early yogis. They belonged to a secret and sacred brotherhood which worshipped the god Rudra (later identified with Shiva) and practised yogic techniques such as Pranayama. They were outcasts (outside the caste system) and even included "untouchables" among their number. The Upanishads, which speak of the direct experience of truth a man can obtain through self-knowledge, were regarded as secret esoteric teachings. Upanishad means literally sitting next to, in other words learning from a teacher. The mystical experience they describe dispenses with superstitious ritual, and hence the need for a priestly class to carry it out.

From the beginning of the Christian era to the Middle Ages, yoga techniques were

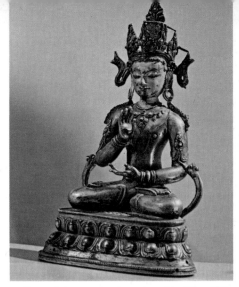

▲ One of the greatest yogis—Buddha. This seventeenth century statue comes from Tibet.

assimilated into many religious schools and sects, nearly always in the form of secret teachings. The Yoga Upanishads, the Tantras and the Hatha Yoga classics use obscure symbolic language and require an initiated teacher to interpret them. For every original work on yoga there are dozens of commentaries. Even in a society which recognizes yoga as a valuable form of self-realization, its practical, experimental nature means that it is best learned from a teacher. A book is best used as a supplementary guide.

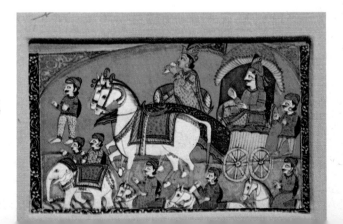

▶ Arjuna with his charioteer, Krishna, ready for battle. The battle forms part of the plot of the epic Mahabharata, in which the Bhagavadgita is set.

Yoga philosophy

The germs of Indian philosophy are in the ancient literature of the Vedas, especially the Upanishads. By the first few centuries AD, six Hindu philosophical systems had been formulated: Vedanta, Samkhya, Yoga, Nyaya, Vaisesika and Mimamsa. Much yoga literature is based on the Vedanta or the Samkhya and Yoga schools, the latter two usually being classed together since their differences are slight.

The systems shared several fundamental ideas. Firstly, that life is full of suffering. This implies that there is something wrong with our form of existence, which may be only a partial picture of the Truth. Secondly, that suffering may be eliminated by obtaining a full knowledge of the Truth. This form of knowledge appears as a direct perception which transcends our everyday consciousness and is reached by looking inwards towards the fundamentals of self. The various ways to self-knowledge are called the yogas. From this it is clear that the Indian concept of philosophy is different from that of the West. Philosophy in India is a means to human progress which is not separate from religion, or from a way of life. There is no one Indian word which corresponds exactly to our word philosophy. The nearest equivalent is Darsana, which means literally sight, in other words perception of Reality. It is this intuitive experience upon which Indian philosophy hinges. It is referred to by many names— Samadhi, Nirvana, Kaivalya, Mukti (liberation)—but in essence it is indescribable. Around this experience has grown up a system of thought with a huge technical vocabulary, both to explain it in terms of philosophy and cosmogony and to attain it

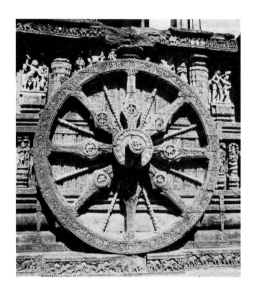

▲ The wheel is a symbol which occurs frequently in Eastern art. It symbolizes the perpetual cycle of existence.

in practical terms. The central experience is common to all the schools of Indian philosophy but the interpretation and terminology vary.

Reincarnation—the Wheel of existence

The cause of man's suffering is said to be ignorance of the nature of the true Self, the spirit in man which is beyond personality and immortal. The Vedanta system calls this ignorance Avidya and the Samkhya Yoga, Aviveka. Whereas the Christian explanation of suffering is punishment for original sin, the Hindus believe that man's true nature is God, but he does not realize it. The

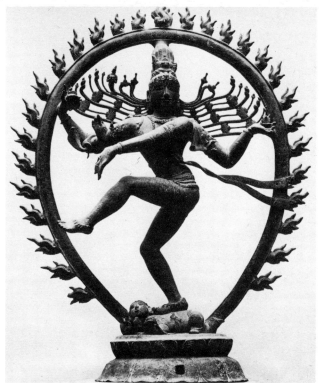

▶ Shiva, representing the life force, worshipped in Saivism, dancing in a circle of fire.

▼ Vishnu the preserver of life, worshipped in Vaisnavism, resting on a coiled snake.

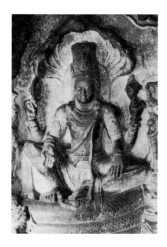

soul is attached to the world by the body as long as it has not realized its true nature. Liberation is only achieved at a stage of spiritual development which most people will not reach within a single lifetime. The soul returns to the world in a new body after death and will continue to do so until it has reached its final stage of evolution. This perpetual cycle is known as the wheel of existence or of Becoming (Samsara) as opposed to the state of Being attained on liberation. For the Hindu, rebirth is not an "afterlife", for the reincarnated soul is still bound to time and its destiny is still to escape from time and rebirth. But it is consoling in the sense that man's progress is in his own hands; after death he has another chance to further himself spiritually.

Karma

Karma means action. It is believed that action determines the soul's progress. The law of Karma is that we reap what we sow, that everyone must suffer the consequences of every action and thought, though the effects may not be immediate. When they occur, the Karma is said to have "ripened". The doctrine of Karma has been interpreted as fatalistic. But while one cannot escape the consequences of past actions (even those who have been enlightened must continue their human life until all past Karma has ripened), the future is determined by the way one acts now. It is believed that the vicious circle may be broken by following the path of yoga.

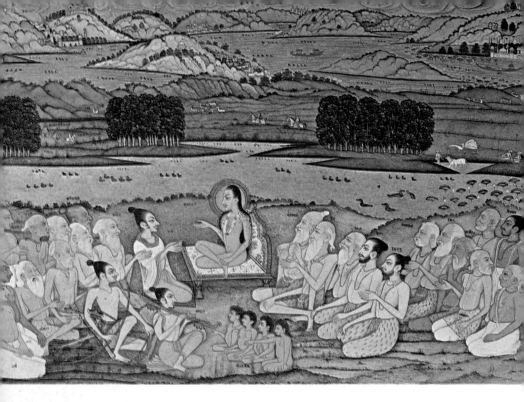

Samkhya yoga

The above ideas are common to all the Hindu systems. The Samkhya Yoga system, which is the philosophy behind the Yoga Sutras by Patanjali, is characterized by its elaborate theory of evolution.

Prakriti is the name given to nature. It consists of three elements, Gunas, which run like threads through the whole of matter. (Guna means rope). The Gunas are: Tamas, the force of darkness and inertia, Rajas, the force of energy, and Sattva, that of light and harmony. The character of a thing is determined by the ratio in which these elements are found in it. In people, Tamas is expressed as ignorance, Rajas as desire and energy, and Sattva as happiness and serenity. The human mind is regarded as of the same stuff as the rest of matter. Before Prakriti became the world, it existed

Buddha teaching his disciples. Buddhism sprang from the same cultural background as the Hindu philosophies. The Buddha himself left no scriptures.

in a formless state, in which the Gunas were in perfect equilibrium. This balance was disturbed by the reflection of the highest Self in Prakriti; the subsequent activity of the Gunas created the world.

Our world is not the only one to have existed; time and again the world is dissolved, withdrawn, then reformed after a period of latency. These dissolutions are called Pralayas. Thus Prakriti is only at work as long as the Spirit identifies itself with it. So, for man to free himself from the constantly changing (and hence suffering) material world, he must reverse the process and dissociate himself from Prakriti by realizing the essential difference between it and his true Self, Purusa. A person's "sense of 'I'" is created by the identification of Purusa with Prakriti. Purusa alone is pure consciousness, beyond the ego and suffering.

Patanjali's Yoga system sets out to refine the stuff of the mind through ethical conduct and meditation until it is pure enough to reflect the Purusa, the real, independent Self. The path to self-knowledge is Vairagya, dispassion, and Abhyasa, practice.

Vedanta

The name Vedanta means "end of the Vedas", in other words, the Upanishads. The central idea of Vedanta is as simple as the Upanishadic statement, "Tatt vam Asi" (Thou art That): everything is one. For the Vedantist there is only one reality, Brahman; the Self (Atman, corresponding to the Purusa of Samkhya) is one facet of Brahman. The world is called Maya, sometimes translated as illusion. For although Brahman is in all things, we do not usually see Brahman in them, but only their outward form. Since Brahman is in everything, by knowing oneself one knows Reality. According to Vedanta, creation is Self-forgetfulness and reality Self-consciousness. Self-forgetfulness is Avidya, the cause of suffering.

Although the Hindu systems differ in theory, they are similar in practice; the goal is liberation and the many yogas form the path.

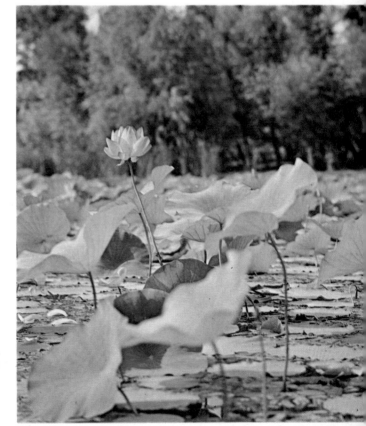

▶ The lotus is a symbol often found in eastern philosophy representing the spiritual development of man. The roots in mud symbolize the physical state, the stem pushing up through the water the intuitive search, and the flower opening in the sunlight spiritual fulfilment.

Types of yoga

There are many types of yoga but they are not opposed. They have been likened to the different strands in a rope. In practice it is impossible to live one kind of yoga without living others. All the yogic paths lead to the same goal and have as their starting point certain basic rules of conduct, known as Yama and Niyama. Yama is a set of commandments prohibiting violence, stealing, covetousness, dishonesty and incontinence. Niyama is a set of observances: purity, austerity, contentment, study and devotion to God. These ten commandments are all positive in spirit. Non-violence, the most important of the Yama, for the others spring from it, is love and compassion for all things. Even if, like Arjuna in the Bhagavadgita, one's duty is to fight, it must be without hate or malice. Contentment is not smugness but a discarding of the superfluous things of life, and of the desire for them, to gain fulfilment from the essentials. Patanjali says: "Contentment brings supreme happiness".

When Samadhi is attained, Yama and Niyama would be observed automatically, for Samadhi is the realization of the oneness of all things, of the good of others as being synonymous with the individual's own good. Before this is experienced, Yama and Niyama are practised as part of the discipline of yoga training, for they help to weaken the egocentric outlook.

The three yogas of the Bhagavadgita

The Bhagavadgita outlines three main paths of yoga, the paths of wisdom, action and devotion: Jnana, Karma, and Bhakti.

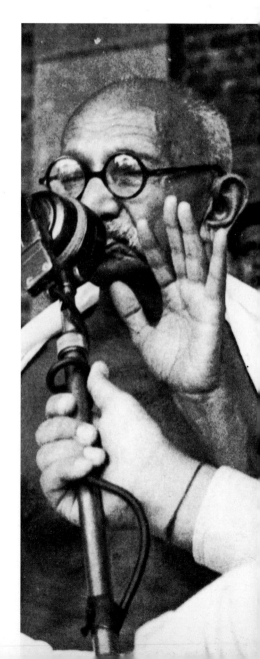

Jnana Yoga is the yoga of knowledge and wisdom. It is practised through reflection, meditation and renunciation. The Jnana yogi is a scholar and an ascetic. His wisdom is described by Krishna thus:

"When one sees Eternity in things that pass away and Infinity in finite things, then one has pure knowledge. But if one merely sees the diversity of things, with their divisions and limitations, then one has impure knowledge. And if one selfishly sees a thing as if it were everything, independent of the One and the many, then one is in the darkness of ignorance."

By understanding with the intellect and meditating on the unity of all things and on the nature of the Self, these truths eventually become self-evident. Intellectual understanding gives way to a direct experience of the Truth.

Karma Yoga is the yoga of action. According to the law of Karma, every action causes more action, and it is impossible to avoid action. The whole of creation is a continually changing process, and even deciding not to act is an act in itself.

"Not by refraining from action does man attain freedom from action. For not even for a moment can a man be without action. Helplessly are all driven to action by the forces born of nature. Great is the man who . . . works on the path of Karma yoga, the path of consecrated action."

Karma yoga is acting dispassionately, detaching oneself from results, not expecting a reward as a right. Actions are performed as offerings, for the good of mankind or the love of God. Every ordinary act is transformed into a kind of sacrifice. The word Karma was originally used in the Vedas to denote the literal sacrifice to the gods.

"He whose undertakings are free from anxious desire and fanciful thought . . . in whatever work he does such a man in truth has peace: he expects nothing, he relies on nothing, and ever has fulness of joy."

◀ Gandhi, a modern yogi who came to epitomize the principle of Ahimsa, non-violence or respect for life. He worked to abolish the Hindu caste system and organized passive resistance to British rule in India.

▶ This diagram illustrates the relationship between different forms of yoga. All yogis start at the rim of the wheel with the ethical rules of Yama and Niyama. All yogic paths lead towards the same goal of spiritual enlightenment at the hub of the wheel.

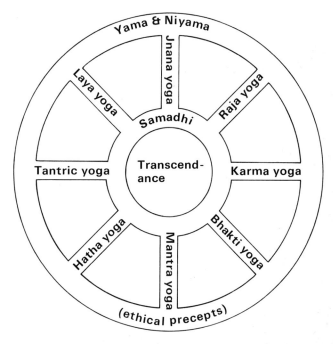

Yama & Niyama
Jnana yoga
Laya yoga
Raja yoga
Samadhi
Tantric yoga
Transcendance
Karma yoga
Hatha yoga
Mantra yoga
Bhakti yoga
(ethical precepts)

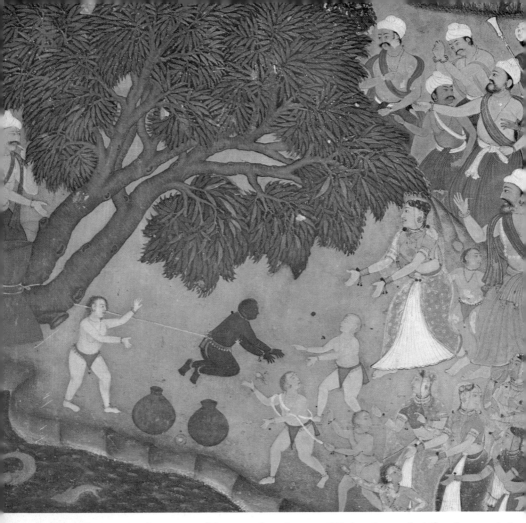

Bhakti Yoga is the yoga of love and devotion and is the third of the great paths outlined in the Bhagavadgita. Knowledge of Brahman through Jnana and Karma yoga is gained only by the wisest and most detached of men: "The path of the Transcendent is hard for mortals to attain."

If a man cannot reach Brahman through wisdom or disinterested action, then he can do so through devotion to God. The god Krishna says:

"To those who adore me with a pure oneness of soul . . . I increase what they have and I give them what they have not. I am the same to all beings and my love is ever the same; but those who worship me with devotion, they are in me and I am in them. For even if the greatest sinner worships me with all his soul, he must be considered righteous . . . For this is my word of promise, that he who loves me shall not perish."

These words are reminiscent of Christ, and the descriptions of Bhakti yoga bear a strong resemblance to the writings of some of the Christian mystics.

16

◀ This painting illustrates a legend about Krishna as a child (shown pulling down the tree). The child Krishna is an object of worship in Bhakti yoga, like the infant Jesus.

▼ A Tibetan mandala or symbolic picture. Mandalas often contain a squared circle, and every detail of the design has spiritual significance.

Tantric yoga

Tantrism was a development in Indian philosophy and practice which appeared around the fourth century AD, grew and flourished in the Middle Ages, and left a strong mark on Indian culture, especially on the visual arts. The philosophy behind Tantrism remains the oneness or non-duality of Vedanta, and spiritual enlightenment, Samadhi, is obtained more by physical means. The yogi uses his own body to induce a mystical experience. The body itself is seen as the temple of the divine, since it houses the Spirit in man, and also because it is regarded as a microcosm of the universe and the gods. The parallels between the body and the cosmos are tapped through ritual practices in order to transcend the normal level of consciousness. Many advanced techniques are used, including the repetition of sacred symbolic sounds (Mantras), the visualization of symbolic imagery (Yantras and Mandalas), the use of light (Trataka), symbolic, ritual gestures (Mudras), and, sometimes as the culmination of a ritual, sexual intercourse (Maithuna).

One of the features of Tantrism is the worship of the female principle represented by the goddess Shakti. For she is the cosmic force itself, the force of creation, and it is through the union of Shakti with Shiva, the male principle and symbol of pure Being, that the duality of the world is transcended and the one eternal Reality apprehended. Tantrism has affinities with alchemy in its experiments towards transmuting the physical into the divine. It was the vehicle for bringing into Hinduism many foreign and exotic elements, especially those of

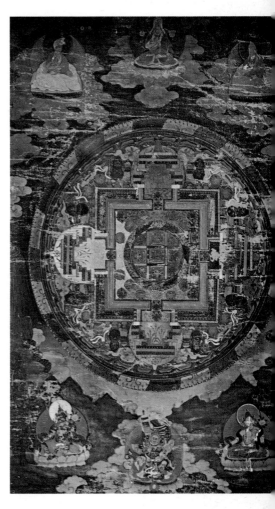

Islam, and for continuing or reviving some ancient and primitive symbols and ritual.

Hatha yoga

Hatha yoga, like Tantric yoga, affects the mind through the body. It consists of

17

cleansing practices and physical exercises used with meditation. The Hatha yoga generally taught in the West is a system of postures (called Asanas) and breathing exercises. Hatha yoga is usually seen as a way of preparing the body and the mind for meditation. But some Hatha techniques are designed to induce Samadhi through direct physical means.

Some of the postures are extremely ancient, and the word Asana is found in the Vedas; but as a complete system, Hatha yoga is a comparatively recent development. The founder of Hatha yoga is said to be a certain Goraksanatha who lived during the first few centuries AD. One of the best known "classics" on Hatha yoga is the Hatha Yoga Pradipika, written in the 15th century. It is allegedly based on a work by Goraksanatha which is now lost. The Pradipika describes fifteen postures; another old text on Hatha yoga, the Siva Samhita, lists more than eighty. These asanas are preliminary exercises designed to make the body a fit vehicle for the powers that will be released in the later stages of training. The power that the yogi learns to experience and control is the life force, the cosmic energy or Prana, which gives life to all things. By a variety of physical and mental techniques, the Hatha yogi succeeds in channelling and concentrating this power to produce an experience of life so intense that it transcends time.

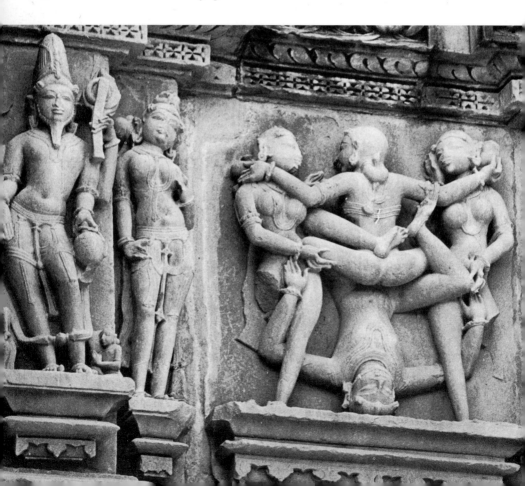

The subtle body

The practice of Hatha yoga is based on a theory of the "subtle body", a kind of invisible parallel to the physical body, in which Prana is generated. It is seen as a network of energy currents which propel the organism. The channels and centres of energy of the subtle body correspond to the physical structure. The central channel, or Nadi, runs through the centre of the spinal column. This is called the Susumma. Two other important Nadis, the Ida and Pingala, run on either side of it, their upper ends being at the openings of the two nostrils.

Centres of energy are called Chakras. There are hundreds of these in the body, but the eight principle Chakras are along the axis of the spine and have a rough but not exact correspondence with the nerve complexes such as the solar plexus. The Chakras have been described as centres of psychic energy, and each of the main Chakras is associated with a different group of bodily functions and a different level of consciousness. By learning to "activate" the Chakras, the yogi achieves deeper and higher levels of awareness than are usually experienced.

The exercises which are designed to stimulate the Chakras and control the flow of Prana are grouped as Asanas, Mudras, and Bandhas, supplemented by Pranayama (breath control). Also, in preparation for these exercises, a number of cleansing and purifying practices are carried out, such as clearing the respiratory tract and cleaning the intestines and bowels. This "unclogging" of the body is done either by passing water or a strip of cloth through the passages, or by special breathing techniques.

The training process of the Hatha yogi gives him extraordinary control over all his human functions. This accounts for the ability of yogis to perform such feats as remaining buried alive for days or weeks or swallowing poison in lethal doses without coming to any harm. These achievements demonstrate the yogi's degree of self-control, but they have no particular value in themselves, being only instrumental in exploring higher states of consciousness. All the physical techniques are accompanied by mental discipline, and the first stage for the Hatha yogi, like any other, is the observance of Yama and Niyama.

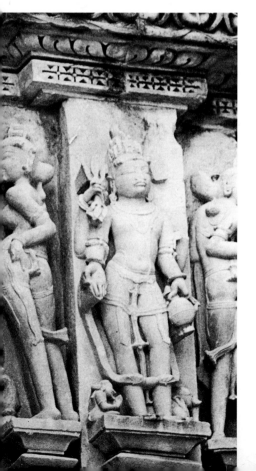

◀ Part of a temple frieze at Khajuraho showing the ritual sex act (Maithuna) which was a feature of Tantric yoga. Far from being an unbridled orgy, it involved self-discipline to the point of withholding semen.

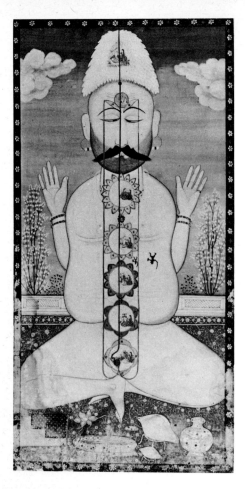

Kundalini yoga

Kundalini is the name of the latent power at the base of the spine, represented by a coiled, sleeping serpent. Most of the Hatha yoga technique described in the Pradipika is intended to "awaken the serpent" and guide it upwards through the central channel of the Susumma, through the centres of the Chakras, to its final goal, the highest Chakra of the brain.

Kundalini has been identified with cosmic energy and with the sexual drive; no one can as yet give a scientific name to it, but there is no doubt that a latent power of some kind exists and can be tapped. The end of Kundalini's journey, union with the highest Chakra, is Samadhi. The techniques used to arouse the force of Kundalini are likened in the literature of Hatha yoga to the effect of beating a snake with a stick. They are very physical, and include movements such as bouncing up and down on the buttocks.

Laya yoga

Laya yoga is a term used to cover Kundalini yoga and the theory of the Chakras. The Chakras are symbolized as lotus flowers with differing numbers of petals; the highest Sahasrara Chakra is the thousand-petalled lotus. Each Chakra has a governing deity. Each is associated, not only with specific moods and functions, but with one of the elements: earth, water, fire, air, ether, consciousness and the divine element. Each has a symbolic visual imagery as well as a symbolic sound, which provide subjects for meditation. The symbology of the Chakras explains the body in terms of a microcosmic representation of the universe —it contains the elements, the gods, the sun and the moon (Ida and Pingala), and the spine as the world's axis. The Hatha yogi thus identifies himself with the cosmos and achieves immortality by transcending the creation of the universe. The union of Kundalini (Shakti) with Shiva in the highest Chakra represents the absorption of the many (the manifold world) into the One (Brahman), or a state of pure Being prior to creation. As the Kundalini rises through the centre of each Chakra, the lotus, whose

▶ This Hatha yogi doing headstand (Sirsasana) comes from a 16th or 17th century Persian manuscript. Some of the 'classical' Asanas have remained unchanged for centuries. Others continue to be adapted according to the needs of different people at different times. The number of yoga postures has grown over the centuries.

One writer on India has said: "too many people in the West think that they are somehow lowering the status of the mind if they admit that it can be influenced by trifling bodily adjustments .. (the Hindus) ... are wiser, they have reared a whole system on these psycho-physical correspondences which to them seem so obvious as to need no discussion."

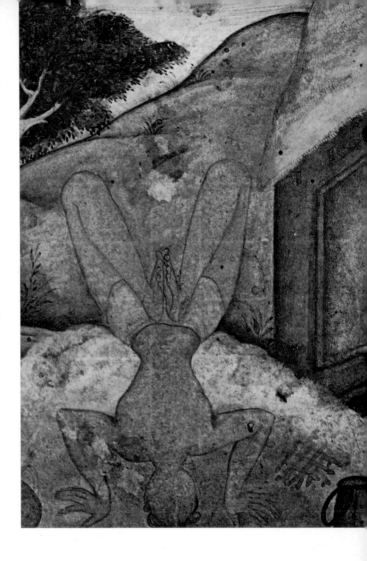

face was turned downwards before, turns upwards, and all the functions associated with that centre are withdrawn, or made latent. Laya yoga means literally the yoga of suspension or absorption. The Hatha Yoga Pradipika says:

"Thus is effected the union of Ida, Pingala, and Susumma (moon, sun and fire) which leads to immortality. The body assumes a deathlike aspect."

In Samadhi all life ceases apart from the state of pure Consciousness. This is the principle of the union of Shiva and Shakti which underlies the sex act in Tantric yoga, the female representing Shakti, the male Shiva. The unification of opposites is the esoteric meaning of Hatha yoga, for "Ha" means sun and "Tha" means moon.

Raja yoga

Raja yoga is the name given to the system of yoga outlined in the Yoga Sutras compiled by Patanjali in about the second century AD. It is also called Astanga yoga, because Astanga means eight limbs or stages, and the Raja yoga path is divided into eight steps. Raja means royal or kingly and Raja yoga involves control of the mind and will. Through meditation awareness is withdrawn from the body, senses and mind, and directed inwards towards the essence of the being. The philosophical background of the Sutras is that of Samkhya. But the Raja yoga technique can be applied within the framework of any philosophy or lifestyle, for the definition of Raja yoga is simply the stilling of the waves of the mind.

The Sutras consist of four books. The first marks out the yogic path in broad terms. The activities of the mind, such as thinking, emoting, dreaming, are classified, and also the human weaknesses which impede progress in meditation: doubt, lethargy, desire, discouragement, etc. Success is achieved through practice (Abhyasa) and detachment (Vairagya). The second book describes the preliminary stages of yoga practice, which prepare for the higher stages of meditation and help to root out the "afflictions" caused by ignorance (Avidya): egoism, desire, aversion and fear. The famous eight limbs are listed. The first two are Yama and Niyama, the ethical rules. The third limb is Asana, posture. This is all that is said on the subject:

"Asana implies steadiness and comfort. It requires relaxation and meditation on the Immovable. Then opposing sensations cease to torment." Meditation is impossible without a comfortable posture.

The fourth limb is Pranayama, breath control. It consists in regulating the in and out breaths, and stopping the breath while the lungs are empty or full. Pranayama

▶ Yogic techniques enable fakirs to perform feats such as sitting on beds of nails without suffering any physical harm. But Patanjali regarded these powers as a danger to spiritual progress.

▼ This picture shows a Brahmin hanging upside down over a fire to demonstrate his devotion to God (Ishvara).

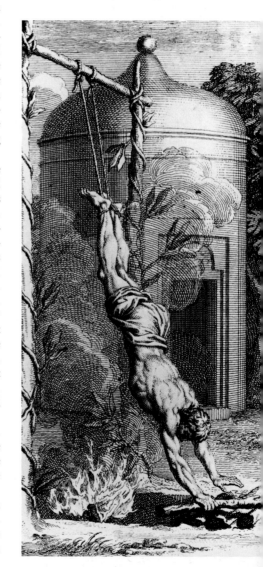

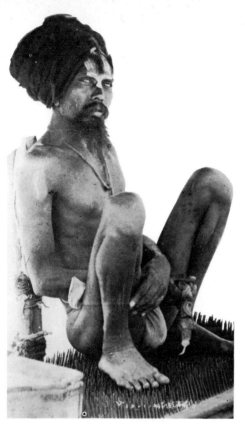

calms and concentrates the mind and body. The fifth limb is Pratyahara, sense withdrawal. This means the detachment of the mind from the objects of the senses. The energy used for sense perception is turned inwards, and used for the practice of the last three limbs of yoga, Dharana (concentration), Dhyana (meditation) and Samadhi. The first five limbs are the outer stages, the last three the inner ones. The last three together are known as Samyama.

The yogi practised in Samyama has developed a powerful instrument he can direct anywhere at will; he is a Siddha, a "perfected one", in possession of occult powers. For example: "By concentration on Udana, living fire, the yogi remains unaffected in water, in swamps or amid thorns; leaves his body at will". But these "supernatural" powers are merely by-products of the yogi's training; in fact they are obstacles to his spiritual progress because they produce temptation.

"These powers of knowledge are obstacles to illumination . . . by renouncing even these powers, the seed of bondage being destroyed, the yogi attains liberation."

Samadhi is not liberation; Samadhi is the

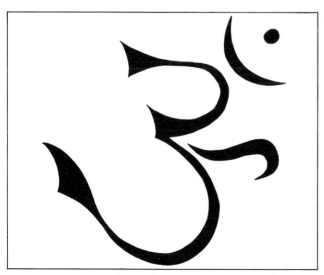

◀ The supreme Mantra, the sacred syllable Om. The three curves represent the physical, mental and supramental states, the dot within the unfinished circle of infinity is the truth or reality which dominates them. Om is common to most eastern countries and may be related to the sound Amen.

23

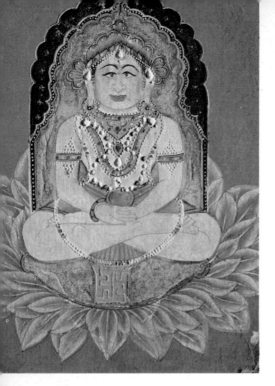

the premature experimentation with advanced yogic techniques. The training process is carefully controlled under the guidance of a teacher, with the emphasis at first almost entirely on the early stages.

Yoga in the West

Few people in the West will be concerned in a practical way with the more esoteric teachings of Classical and Hatha yoga. The yoga that is becoming increasingly relevant to our way of life is that of relaxation and meditation, a combination of Hatha yoga postures and Raja yoga. The two can no more be separated than can the body from the mind, and it is the application of yoga as a psychotherapeutic technique which is now helping people to keep sane and healthy in the modern world. The yoga postures not only keep the body supple and healthy but they directly affect the mind and emotions. For it is believed that every part of the body has psychological significance and that every psychological activity is expressed by the attitudes and moods of the body. For example, a mentally downtrodden attitude may be expressed as a stooping posture with hunched shoulders. Adjusting the posture to an upright, relaxed, open one influences the psychological attitude.

Hindu philosophers have never recognized a qualitative difference between mind and body. Both are composed of the same elements of matter or energy, the mind being a more refined form of matter. Western science now acknowledges that there is no clear demarcation between the two. Bodily posture, breathing and sense

ultimate refining of the mind, through meditation, so that it can reflect the Self with total clarity. Then even the practice of Samadhi is discarded and liberation achieved. The yogi is released from the world process; after his death he will not be reborn. "Then action and affliction come to an end. The procession of Qualities (Gunas) comes to an end; their purpose is fulfilled".

The most advanced stages of Hatha and Raja yoga involve the rechannelling of energy inwards towards an intense inner experience. Our energy is normally dispersed in many ways—through physical activity, the stimulation of the senses, thought, emotion, sexual experience (Kundalini yoga may be the sublimation of sexual energy)—and when it is concentrated it has a tremendous destructive as well as creative power. Hence the warnings that are sounded in books on yoga against

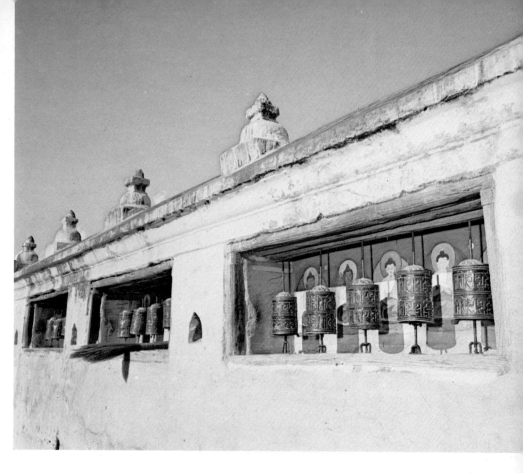

impressions are controlled by the mind and in turn affect the mind. B.K.S. Iyengar, in his book *Light on Yoga,* says:

"Hatha and Raja yoga complement each other and form a single approach towards Liberation".

Mantra yoga

Mantra Yoga is the repetition of meaningful sounds as an aid to meditation. Mantras have the same creative power as prayers or spells. They are basic syllables based on the sounds of the different vibrations of energy which make up the universe. The theory behind the Mantra is that forms arise from sound ("In the beginning was the Word"), forms are affected by sound, and every movement gives rise to a sound, even if it is beyond our hearing. Thus, for every form there is a corresponding sound. Each of the Chakras (energy centres) in the body has its own basic syllable, called its "seed Mantra". Uttering its sound evokes the power associated with it. The Mantra can be compared with the chanting of prayers, such as the Hail Mary or the Lord's Prayer. Of course, like prayers, Mantras are ineffective unless uttered with intention and conviction. Repetition of the right Mantra with intense concentration is said to induce Samadhi.

Yoga and science

As the frontiers of the sciences are pushed forward, so the barriers between them become more artificial. For the yogi such barriers have never existed. Philosophy, religion, astrology, physics, psychology, are all interrelated.

Yoga and physics

Modern physics is discovering that matter is not as solid and permanent as was once assumed. There is proportionately as much space inside the atom as there is in the universe. Moreover, the "particles" in atoms are not themselves solid, but consist of waves of electromagnetic action. Matter is a form of energy, an idea which was commonplace to Indian philosophers more than two thousand years ago.

Fundamental to the Samkhya philosophy is the idea that matter can be neither created nor destroyed. Organic and inorganic forms are produced by constant rearrangement of basic elements. All things on earth are united by their basic similarity in structure and function. Just as there is no clear demarcation between inorganic and organic matter, so it is impossible to distinguish absolutely between body and mind.

The physiology of yoga

Medical research has confirmed the beneficial effects of yoga postures on the body. Spine and joints are kept flexible (yoga can prevent and alleviate osteoarthritis), the whole metabolism is stimulated and the body's healing powers improved. The stretching and compressing which take place in yoga exercises, and the alteration of the body's orientation and centre of gravity (for example in the shoulder stand) have been shown to generate piezo-electricity in the body tissues (electricity caused by pressure). Regular piezo-electric charges regulate the growth, maintenance and strengthening of connective tissue, help the passage of nutrients through the cell walls and accelerate healing and the production of white cells and antibodies.

Laboratory tests have demonstrated the ability of yogis to control voluntarily the autonomic or involuntary functions of the body, such as pulse, blood pressure and activity of internal organs and glands, and a system known as biofeedback has been invented to teach people how to achieve

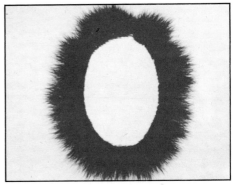

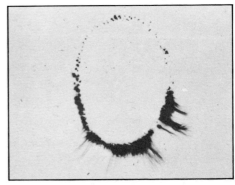

this control quite quickly. This has obvious applications in treating high blood pressure, for example. Biofeedback is also used to enable people to achieve mental states associated with meditation. Electroencephalograph measurements have shown that during meditation the brain emits a high proportion of Alpha waves. These are related to a relaxed, tensionless state of mind, a passive awareness in which the rational mind and the senses are inoperative. Alpha waves are also associated with creativity. The research done so far indicates that meditation can prevent and cure psychosomatic disorders.

Yoga and psychology

Since Jung wrote a psychological commentary on an ancient Chinese text in 1929 there has been increasing interest in the comparison between Western psychotherapy and Eastern philosophy. There are similarities between psychoanalysis and the earlier stages of yoga practice. Both aim to integrate the human being by harmonizing his separate functions and bringing him into harmony with the world around him. The disturbed person often suffers from alienation, a heightened sense of his individual separateness. Yoga emphasizes the relationship between the individual and the rest of society and the universe (and hence his sense of value as an essential part of the scheme). Both Yoga and psychoanalysis work on the principle of self-knowledge or an understanding of the way in which the mind works, through experience. Both see compulsive and automatic (or conditioned) behaviour as negative and destructive and try to free the self from the tensions which cause it.

▶ The physical effects of meditation being tested in the laboratory. Here the subject is screened so that his observations do not affect his performance, but the instruments can be used to help people to attain states of meditation.

◀ These photographs were taken by a special camera which reveals the energy emitted by objects and people. They show the finger of a person early in the morning (above) and again in the evening (below). Yogis have often been able to perceive other people's "auras" and to assess from them their degree of vitality.

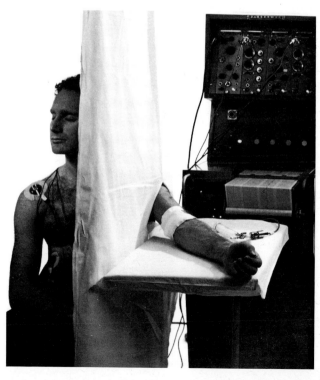

Yoga today

One does not have to be a Hindu to practise yoga. Christians and atheists can be yogis. It has been said that yoga makes you a better exponent of whatever lifestyle; for yoga relaxes the hold on conditioned habits and ways of thinking which limit a view of the world and your own potential. Yoga is a practice which develops the potential that is in every human being.

Most people who take up yoga in the West today probably do so not to achieve spiritual enlightenment but to learn to relax. The yoga postures are a marvellous method of physical exercise and relaxation. But it soon becomes apparent that physical tension is closely related to mental tension.

The performance of the postures demands and produces concentration and stilling of the mind, not only because you must concentrate in order to do them, but because certain physical postures are expressive of mental states. A simple example is the reflection of mental tension in a tense neck and shoulders.

Yoga works on the whole person. The Bhagavadgita says: "Yoga is a harmony." Yoga harmonizes the parts of the body; body and mind; the individual and the outside world. For yoga stresses the relationships between all things rather than the divisions. A person does not end with his outer layer of skin but touches every-

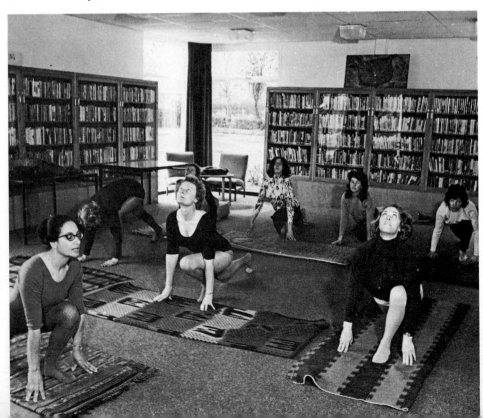

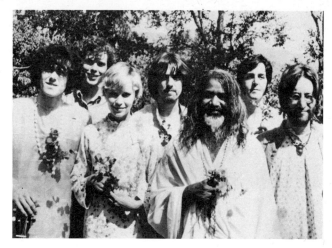

► The Maharishi Mahesh Yogi with some of his Western disciples at his Ashram in the Himalayas. His Transcendental Meditation technique, based on the use of a personal Mantra, has become popular in Europe and America.

thing around him, just as the shape of objects is defined by the space around them. Every breath, every action, every thought, affects the environment. Many people see themselves as small, separate units in an alien world, clinging to their identity and feeling helplessly insignificant. Most of us do not even see things clearly because our perception is coloured by per-

sonal desires, anxieties and prejudices.

In meditation, the mind is cleared of egocentric thoughts and emotions, and just looks, whether at an object or at the mind. By learning to look, and accept, with-

◄ A yoga class in London. More and more people are taking up yoga, usually with the motive of learning how to relax.

▼ The hydrogen bomb. One of the principles of yoga is that all matter is energy. and that huge amounts of energy are latent in matter. One of the aims of yoga practice is to release the potential energy in the human being.

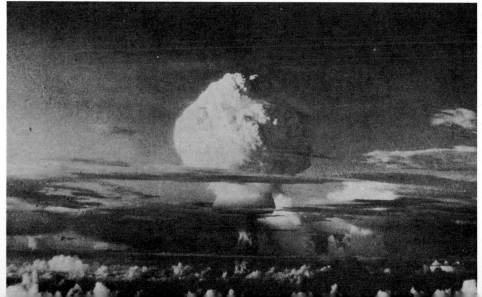

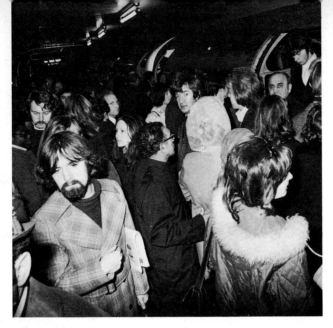

out judgement, one becomes receptive to the true nature of things, including oneself. Then the relationships between things become apparent. Swami Satyananda Saraswati says:

"If our mind is reasonably untroubled and loving, then we will see the environment in the same light. If our mind is habitually relaxed, then we will see the world in a similar way, where everything is harmonious." Some people are alarmed at the idea of losing their sense of ego, imagining that their individuality will be submerged in a kind of nothingness. But to see the world as a harmonious whole is not to lose personal individuality. The hand is a part of the body with a very individual function, but its usefulness depends upon its being an integral part: cut it off and it is useless. Hence the emphasis in yoga on knowing oneself, through yoga practice, and simply doing your own work to the best of your ability. If work is carried out in the spirit of Karma yoga, with a purpose, but without attachment to the results, this leads to an equanimity which enables one to "do what one has to do" without resentment or a sense of frustration or failure. The Gita says:

"Greater is thine own work, even if this be humble, than the work of another, even if this be great."

And in the words of Ernest Wood in his book on yoga:

"One need not seek outside one's own small personal existence for the greater, unlimited opportunity. With this realization comes the final death of greed, of hating, of fanaticism, of self-satisfaction, and of stupidity."

Yoga is an antidote to the "rat-race", for it is essentially non-competitive. Each person knows his own achievements in relation to his own abilities and need not judge his work by external standards. In yoga there can be no failure as long as there is trying. Patanjali says: "Success is immediate where effort is intense" and Krishna says to Arjuna:

"Hear now the wisdom of Yoga, path of the Eternal and freedom from bondage. No step is lost on this path, and no dangers are found. And even a little progress is freedom from fear." One can start anywhere in yoga and benefit from it, for yoga is not simply a means to an end but a way of life.

There are many concrete physical benefits of yoga, that are felt as soon as one starts regular practice. Yoga keeps one healthy, since it helps respiration, digestion, elimination and circulation. It keeps the body supple, stretches the spine and strengthens the muscles. Minor ailments and psychosomatic symptoms often disappear. All this creates a general feeling of well-being, a physical lightness and buoyancy, and a feeling of being at one with things. You usually become more aware of your surroundings since yoga stimulates the entire organism, making one more "alive". Whatever a person's problem, whether it is over-eating, smoking, or any other form of compulsive behaviour, yoga can help by restoring the balance between the natural functions of the body and those of the mind. With regular practice, the yogi becomes in tune with himself and may find himself adjusting habits such as diet, clothing and fixed routine; and cutting down on the props of life, from smoking, drinking and over-eating to the more superfluous material acquisitions.

"Yoga is a harmony. Not for him who eats too much, or for him who eats too little; not for him who sleeps too little, or for him who sleeps too much. When . . . he is master of his own inner life . . . then he is called a yogi in harmony. To him, gold or stones or earth are one. He has risen on the heights of his soul. And in peace he beholds relatives, companions and friends, those impartial or indifferent or who hate him: he sees them all with the same inner peace."

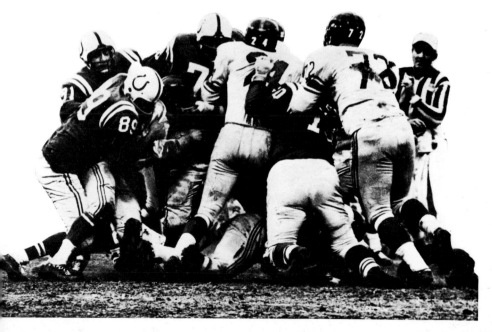

Preparing for action

Place and time

1. A clean, quiet, airy place is ideal for yoga. If you can, practise outdoors in the summer. **2.** Early morning and evening are good times to practise. In the morning you may feel fresh and energetic, but will be stiff. In the evening you will feel looser but you may be tired. You could divide your practice between the two times of day, since some postures are conducive to sleep.

Clothes and equipment

3. Clothes should be completely unrestricting. **4.** Feet should be bare, so that they have freedom of movement and make firm contact with the ground. When it is warm it is best to wear as few clothes as possible. **5.** The only "equipment" you need is a blanket or rug for the sitting and lying postures.

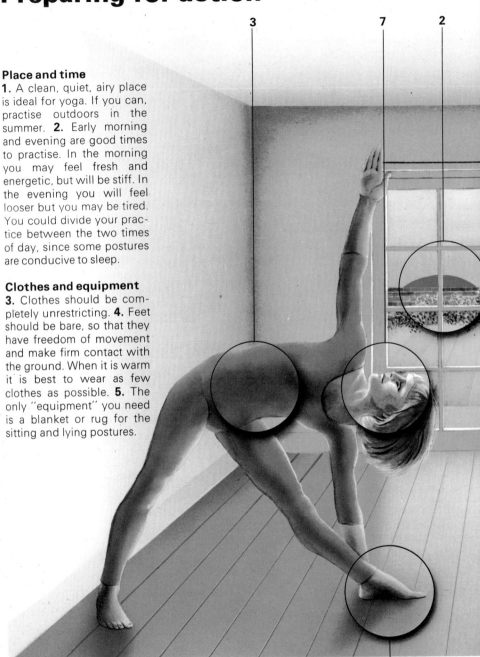

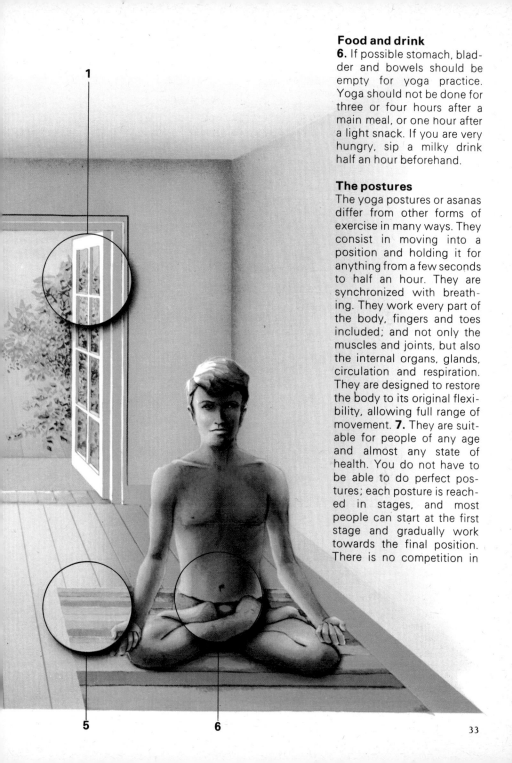

Food and drink

6. If possible stomach, bladder and bowels should be empty for yoga practice. Yoga should not be done for three or four hours after a main meal, or one hour after a light snack. If you are very hungry, sip a milky drink half an hour beforehand.

The postures

The yoga postures or asanas differ from other forms of exercise in many ways. They consist in moving into a position and holding it for anything from a few seconds to half an hour. They are synchronized with breathing. They work every part of the body, fingers and toes included; and not only the muscles and joints, but also the internal organs, glands, circulation and respiration. They are designed to restore the body to its original flexibility, allowing full range of movement. **7.** They are suitable for people of any age and almost any state of health. You do not have to be able to do perfect postures; each posture is reached in stages, and most people can start at the first stage and gradually work towards the final position. There is no competition in yoga; every person works to extend his own limitations, and an elderly or stiff person may derive greater personal benefit from working in the early stages than a supple person who can sit in a lotus posture effortlessly.

The slow, rhythmical movements in yoga are important. Loosening up is achieved by working to the limit of one's movement and holding there, not by jerking into position. It is at the extremes of movement that the greatest weakness lies, and yoga strengthens the body at these points, contributing to an overall feeling of strength and well-being.

The systematic nature of yoga ensures that all sides (front, back; left, right; top, bottom) are worked evenly. This leads to symmetrical posture and correct full breathing. Some postures, when completed, are relaxed positions, suitable for meditation, though it may take months or more of practice to reach the relaxed stage. Other postures are dynamic, and some are surprisingly strenuous. It is important never to force the body, and to be aware of your own limits, which should be extended gradually.

The spine
Although the postures tone up the entire body, one of their chief features is the way in which they work the spine. The spine supports the body and the weight of the head, and also houses part of the central nervous system. A strong flexible back helps one to stay healthy. In yoga all parts of the spine are stretched, bent forwards and back, and twisted laterally.

A few cautions
Unlike many other forms of exercise, you do not have to be very fit, strong, or supple to benefit from yoga, though regular practice should make you all of these things. Many people start yoga who are not used to physical exercise, so if you are one of these, take it gently to begin with. As soon as the discomfort of unaccustomed stretching becomes the pain of strain, stop. Stop if there is undue strain in the face, ears, eyes or breathing. Anyone suffering from a specific problem such as an adverse heart condition or detached retina should consult his doctor or an experienced yoga teacher. There are beneficial postures for almost every condition, but also some which should be avoided. Women should not practise the upside-down postures during menstruation. Yoga can be practised for the first three months of a normal pregnancy, and for longer if one is unusually fit.

Breathing
Always breathe through the nose if possible when practising the postures. Normally, a movement requiring effort is done on an exhalation, with a deep inhalation immediately before it. The most important thing is never to hold the breath. When in doubt about the breathing, breathe normally.

Names of the postures
Most of the postures are named after gods, people, animals and plants (warrior, camel, serpent, locust, tree, etc.). This reflects the philosophy that the universal spirit is in all things; the yogi assumes the forms of all things in nature while practising the asanas. The Brihadaranyaka Upanishad says: "The Atman (spirit) in man is the very same as the vital force in the elephant, the gnat, the ant, the four quarters of the world; in short, the Atman in man is part and parcel of the whole universe."

Postures in this book
The postures in this book are divided into twenty basic postures and a group of additional postures, mostly more advanced. All the asanas are based on the teaching of B. K. S. Iyengar.

Beginners are advised to practise the standing postures regularly, since they are a vital preparation for any more advanced work.

Remember that any posture which works one side of the body should be repeated on the other. Always read through all the instructions for a pose before you start to do it.

The effect of the asanas on the mind is relaxing. Iyengar says, "it is the body alone which should be active while the brain should remain passive, watchful and alert." After every yoga session, however short, relax in Savasana (corpse pose) for a few minutes.

Tadasana—*mountain*

Tadasana is the basic standing posture. When practising the other standing postures, Tadasana is the position one returns to in between. Although it is a simple posture, there are many points to bear in mind until it becomes a habit. It is very important to practise this position because it brings awareness of the way one stands and improves posture generally. Bad posture leads to physical and mental fatigue. This is a good position in which to practise deep breathing.

Stand upright with feet together and parallel, heels and big toes touching. Be aware of both feet in even contact with the floor, and of some weight on the heels.

Tighten the knees by pulling up the kneecaps, stretching the back of the thighs.

Stretch the spine from its base to the crown of the head. The shoulders should be down and relaxed, think of them as being like a clothes hanger, with the arms and hands hanging loosely from them. If the chest is open the hands will hang slightly away from the thighs.

Do not hollow the back or let the stomach stick out. Expand the chest. Pull up the back of the neck and head so that the chin does not jut out but is slightly tucked in. It is the crown of the head which should be uppermost.

Make sure that your weight is evenly balanced on your feet, so that you are not tilting forward onto your toes or backwards onto the heels. This ensures that the spine is pulled up in the correct, natural position. When the body weight is unevenly distributed on the feet, this puts strain on the spine.

Points to watch
Have the feet parallel, with big toes together.
Pull the knees tight.
Pull the stomach in.
Stretch the spine.
Relax the shoulders.
Relax the hands.
Open the chest, drop the shoulders back.
Relax the face and throat.
Imagine a string attached to the crown of the head, like a puppet, gently pulling the body up.

Uttihita Trikonasana—*triangle*

The triangle pose stretches the legs, back and neck and helps to loosen the hips. Many of the standing postures make the hips more supple and are thus a good preparation for the cross-legged positions such as the lotus, which are often difficult for Western people. Trikonasana involves a bend sideways from the hips. This means that the hips must not turn so that the body twists, but must be kept facing forwards throughout. A good way of ensuring this is to do the posture standing with your back to a wall.

Stand in Tadasana. Spread the feet 1 metre apart. Turn the right foot out 90 degrees to the right, and turn the left foot in slightly.

Breathe in and raise the arms sideways to shoulder level. Exhale, bending to the right, sliding the right hand down towards the floor. Look up at the left thumb. Breathe normally, holding the position, then breathe in while standing up. Repeat to the left. Relax.

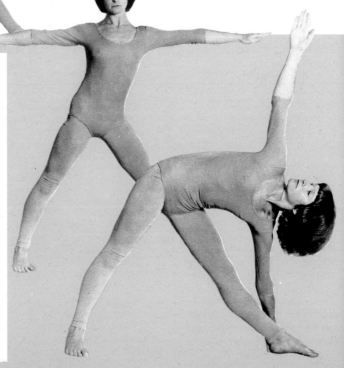

Points to watch
Don't try to put your hand on the floor at the expense of turning the hips. If necessary, rest the lower hand on the leg.

Try to extend the body while bending, pulling the ribs sideways before going down.

When raising the arms before bending sideways, keep the shoulders down.

In the completed position, stretch the arms. Stretch the back of the neck while turning the head to look at the upper hand.

Keep the knees pulled tight throughout.

Uttihita Parsvakonasana

Uttihita means stretched. Parsva means side. Kona means angle. This posture produces a powerful stretch all along the straight side of the body. At first it feels strange and uncomfortable, but when you are used to practising it, you welcome the invigorating feeling of stretch. Like Trikonasana, this posture consists of a sideways bend in which the hips must face squarely forward.

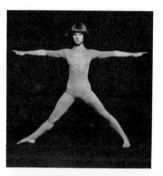 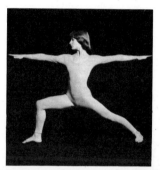

Stand in Tadasana, then space the feet $1\frac{1}{2}$ metres apart. Turn the right foot out 90 degrees to the right and the left foot in slightly.

Breathe in and raise the arms to shoulder level, without lifting the shoulders. As you breathe out, bend the right knee until the right shin is vertical to the floor. Keep the bent knee pressed back and the straight knee pulled up tight.

Now take another breath, and as you breathe out, bend sideways to the right, dropping the right hand to the floor, or, if it won't reach, bend it and rest the lower arm just above the right knee. The left arm should be stretched alongside the left ear, with the palm facing the floor.

Turn the head to look up in front of the outstretched left arm. Experience the strong pull along the left side, stretching from heel to fingertips.

Breathe normally while holding the pose, then breathe in as you stand up. Bring the feet together and repeat on the other side.

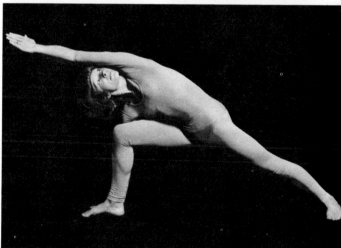

Points to watch
Check the position of the bent leg. The thigh should be parallel to the floor if possible, and the shin vertical. The knee should be directly above the ankle.
Keep the back leg quite straight. Try the pose against a wall, keeping the upper shoulder, hip and bent knee pressed towards it.

Virabhadrasana I —*warrior*

This posture and the one on the opposite page are named after a legendary warrior hero called Virabhadra.
The first posture, Virabhadrasana I, is quite strenuous and should not be held too long. Do not attempt it if you have a weak heart, high blood pressure or palpitations. This posture expands the chest, strengthens the legs and back, and makes the back and shoulders supple. The second posture, Virabhadrasana II, stretches and strengthens the leg and back muscles. Practice of these standing postures prepares the body for the later forward bending movements since they strengthen and loosen the back and the pelvic area.

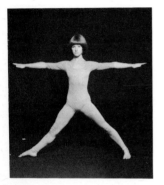

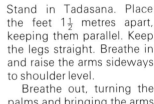

Stand in Tadasana. Place the feet 1½ metres apart, keeping them parallel. Keep the legs straight. Breathe in and raise the arms sideways to shoulder level.

Breathe out, turning the palms and bringing the arms straight above the head. Now turn the right foot 90 degrees to the right and the left foot about 60 degrees to the right, turning the whole body with the feet. Keep the legs straight. Try to keep your arms straight and shoulders down. Bring the palms together and pull the arms back behind your ears. You may find that this may not

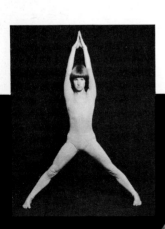

Virabhadrasana II

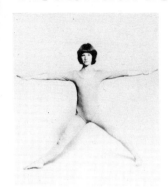

Stand in Tadasana. Spread the feet 1½ metres apart; turn the right foot 90 degrees to the right and the left foot in slightly.

Breathe in and stretch the arms sideways. As you breathe out, bend the right knee until the thigh is horizontal and the shin vertical Breathe normally and turn the head to the right. Breathe in as you straighten the right knee and repeat on the left.

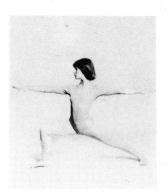

be possible at first: the important thing is to keep the arms straight and avoid lifting the shoulders.

Take a breath in, and as you breathe out, bend the right knee until the shin is vertical to the floor. The right thigh should be horizontal, the right knee directly above the ankle. Concentrate on keeping the back leg absolutely straight, with the knee pulled tight. Breathe evenly as you hold this position, and don't hold it too long. Breathe in as you straighten the right leg. Drop the arms, then repeat the exercise on the other side.

Points to watch

Make sure the bent knee does not roll forward or bend beyond the foot as shown below.

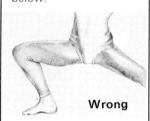

Wrong

The face, chest and right knee should face the same way as the right foot.
The back foot should be flat on the floor.
The weight should not be on the inner edges of the feet.
Do not raise the shoulders.
Keep the arms straight. Relax the front of the body, face and throat and diaphragm, it is the back which is working.

Uttanasana—*relaxed*

This posture is a relaxing one and can be done between the other standing postures, especially the more strenuous ones, in order to relax the body and refresh the mind. It has a very soothing effect. This posture is also helpful in preparing the body for the sitting forward bends since it uses gravity to pull the upper body down from the hips. Not suitable for anyone with a slipped disc.

Stand in Tadasana. Make sure the spine is well stretched without hollowing the back or sticking out the stomach. Take a deep breath in, then on the out breath bend forward from the hips. Keep the back straight as you bend forwards, leading with the chest. Keep the head up so that you are looking straight ahead of you until you have completed the bending movement, then drop the head and let it relax completely. Now breathe normally. Concentrate on keeping the knees pulled tight and at the same time relaxing the upper body. You will feel your own weight gradually pulling you lower. Hold this position as long as you like, then stand up while you breathe in, lifting the head first and keeping the back straight.

Points to watch
Keep the back straight as you bend forward and stand up again. When in position, let the upper body hang as limply as a rag doll; concentrate especially on relaxing the head and neck.

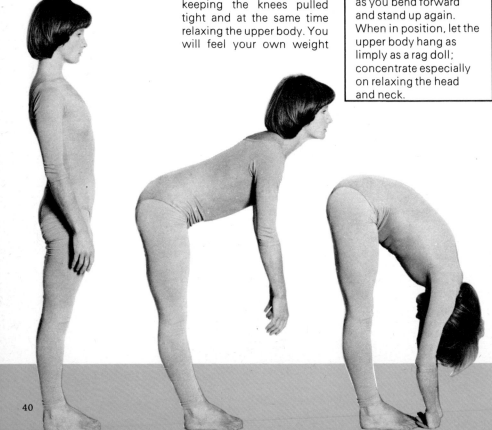

Vrksasana—*tree*

This posture requires stability, balance and concentration. If at first you find it impossible not to wobble, then try doing it with your back against a wall. The supporting leg should be pulled tight at the knee so that it feels very stable, with the foot planted firmly on the ground. It will help you to balance if you fix your gaze on a spot in the distance.

Stand in Tadasana. Bend the right knee, take the right foot in both hands and place it firmly against the opposite thigh, toes pointing downwards. Press the sole of the foot well into the left thigh.

Now stand very tall, with the left leg absolutely straight. Place the palms of your hands together and slowly raise the arms until they are straight above the head. Try not to let the shoulders lift with the arms. Gently press the bent knee back.

Breathe deeply while you hold the pose for a few seconds, then release the arms and leg and stand again in Tadasana. Repeat the pose standing on the right leg.

Points to watch
If you tighten the muscles in the supporting leg and press the sole of the other foot firmly into the thigh, you will find it easier to balance.
Try not to let the bent knee roll forwards.

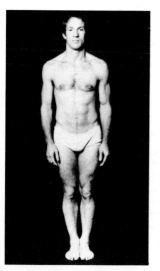

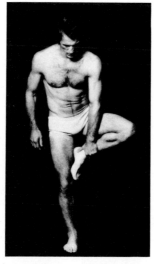

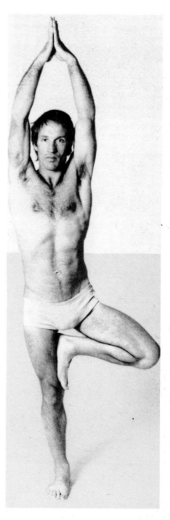

Parsvottanasana

This posture consists of a sequence of movements. The position of the hands behind the back stretches the wrists, making the wrist joints more flexible. It also opens the chest, for it pushes the shoulders back and the chest forward. This facilitates deeper breathing and corrects rounded shoulders in everyday posture. The two-way bending of the back makes the spine supple, and the turning of the feet combined with the forward bend also reduces stiffness in the hip muscles. The posture is quite difficult for many people to begin with but it is worth persevering, for it gives one a very good 'feel' of how the body should stand and move.

Stand in Tadasana. Place the palms of the hands together behind the back, fingers pointing downwards. Draw the shoulders and elbows back. Now turn the wrists so that the fingers point upwards along the centre of the back, with the fingers on a level with the shoulder blades. If this is comfortable, proceed with the posture in this position.

If the position of the hands is very uncomfortable, or if you cannot do it at all, continue the posture with the hands holding the elbows behind the back.

Place the feet 1 metre apart. Turn the right foot 90 degrees and the left foot about 60 degrees to the right. Keep the legs quite straight throughout. Take a breath in and drop the head back so that you are looking directly above you and so that the top of the back bends slightly. As you breathe out, bend forward from the hips, keeping the back straight. The movement should be similar to the forward bend shown on page 40.

Points to watch
Keep the knees pulled tight throughout.
Keep your elbows pressed back.
Keep the throat relaxed.

After releasing the hands, do not shake them but turn them away from the body and gently move the fingers to ease stiffness.

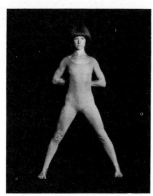

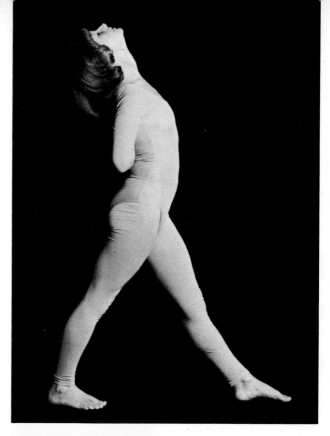

Relax the neck, letting the head drop towards the right knee. Stay in this pose with normal breathing for up to twenty seconds, then turn both feet until they are pointing in the reverse direction, swinging the body around to the left. As you breathe in, lift the body up and drop the head as far back as possible, keeping the legs straight. Breathe out as you bend forward again, dropping the head down.

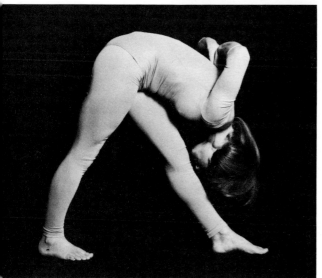

After holding this pose with normal breathing, swivel the feet until they are facing forward and parallel, moving the head to the centre. Then breathe in as you stand up straight. Release the hands.

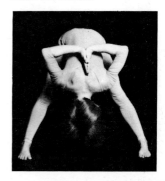

Shoulder exercise

This exercise is not a complete posture in itself. It is part of a more difficult pose in which the leg movement may not be possible at first. On its own it is a very good exercise for loosening the shoulders. Many people have very stiff shoulders through bad posture and through mental tension. The neck and shoulders are areas where tension frequently sets in. These loosening-up exercises help one to become aware of tension when it is present and to consciously relax.

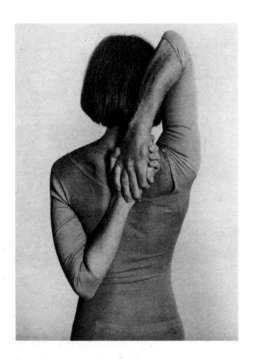 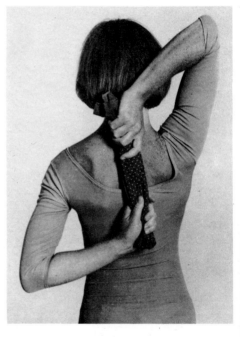

Stand in Tadasana. Breathe in and raise the right arm above the head, bringing the left hand up the centre of the back. As you breathe out, reach the hands together and clasp them.

If your hands will not meet, use a cloth as shown in the picture. Try to wriggle the hands nearer to each other. If you can catch the hands easily, try to hold the wrists.

Release the hands, relax the arms, then repeat the exercise on the other side.

You may find a surprising difference in the mobility of your two shoulders. This illustrates the imbalance that exists in almost everyone, that yoga helps to correct.

Dandasana—*staff*

Danda means a staff or rod. The back should be completely straight in this posture. It is deceptively simple, for many adults find that the back muscles must work very hard to maintain the position. This weakness comes from a lifetime of sitting in chairs. It is interesting to see how easily a very young child assumes this position and holds it quite comfortably.

Points to watch
When the back is well pulled up, it forms a right angle with the legs.
Beginners should do the position against a wall.

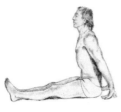

Sit on the floor on your yoga mat or rug, with your legs stretched straight out in front of you. Make sure you are sitting well forward on the bones of the pelvis, not rolling backwards on to the base of the spine.

Place your hands on the floor beside your hips, the fingers pointing towards your feet. If your arms are not very long, place the tips of the fingers on the floor. Use your arms to help push the chest forward and straighten the back. Hold the position only as long as you can without strain, then relax and repeat two or three times.

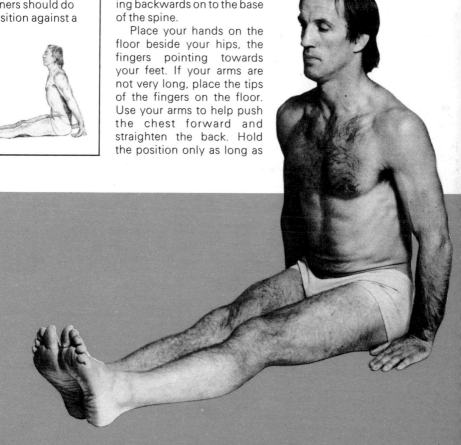

Paschimottanasana—*forward bend*

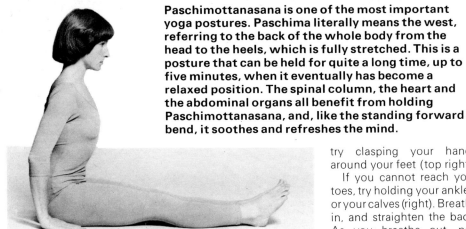

Paschimottanasana is one of the most important yoga postures. Paschima literally means the west, referring to the back of the whole body from the head to the heels, which is fully stretched. This is a posture that can be held for quite a long time, up to five minutes, when it eventually has become a relaxed position. The spinal column, the heart and the abdominal organs all benefit from holding Paschimottanasana, and, like the standing forward bend, it soothes and refreshes the mind.

try clasping your hands around your feet (top right). If you cannot reach your toes, try holding your ankles, or your calves (right). Breathe in, and straighten the back. As you breathe out, pull

First (above) sit in Dandasana. Press the backs of the knees to the floor to straighten the legs. Pull the back up straight, with chest forward and shoulders back. Do not point the feet, but keep them relaxed.

Now reach forward (right) with your hands and slide them down your legs to a place where you can hold them comfortably without rounding the shoulders. If you cannot reach your toes, see the opposite page for alternative positions. Now take in a deep breath, at the same time straightening the back and keeping the chest open. As you breathe out (right), extend the back and pull yourself forward from the hips, attempting to stretch the ribcage flat along the legs. If you can rest your body along your legs, drop your head down and touch your face on to your knees. When you can do this easily,

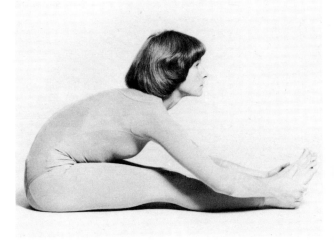

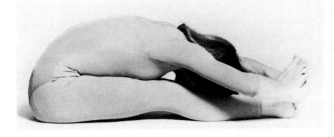

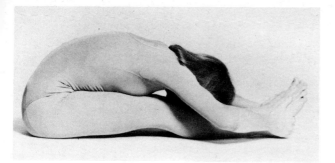

yourself forward as far as you can (below right), bending from the hips. If you find that you have very little movement in the hips, see the alternative method below.

Breathe normally while you hold the position. Don't hold it for too long at first, but build up the time gradually. Try holding, then relaxing, then holding again. If you wish to extend the back further while in position, do so gently on an out breath.

If you are extremely stiff in the hips and lower back, use a towel or a belt (below) to loop around your feet. Use this to pull yourself forward, keeping the shoulders down

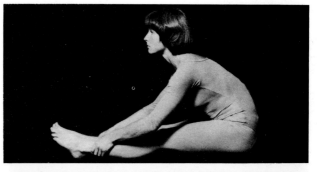

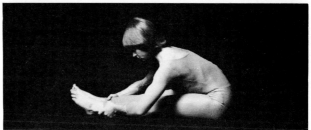

and the chest forward. Don't despair if you hardly bend at all; the loosening-up process is a very gradual one. If you practise it regularly, and if you also practise the standing postures, you will eventually make progress. It is the work you are doing now which is important, not the results.

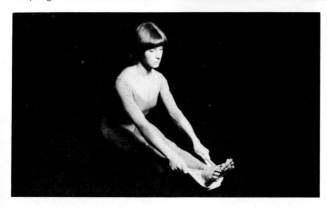

Janu Sirsasana

This posture consists of a forward bend along one outstretched leg. As in Paschimottanasana, the head eventually rests on the knee. Janu means knee and Sirsa means head. The other knee is bent and pulled back. Janu Sirsasana stimulates the internal organs and improves digestion. It especially tones the kidneys, and the effect of this can be felt in the lower back while bending forward. Most people find that they can bend forward more easily in this posture than in Pachimottanasana, the full forward bend.

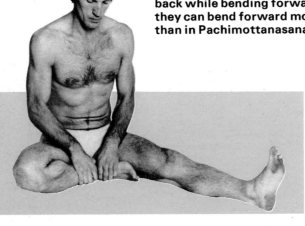

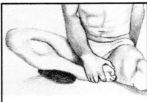

Points to watch
Keep the knee of the straight leg pressed down against the floor. Keep the bent knee pushed back.
Don't 'hump' the back when you bend forward. It is better to keep the head up if you can't bend very far.
If it is painful to keep the leg bent without support, wedge a blanket or cushion under the thigh (see above).

Sit in Dandasana. Bend the right knee and draw the right foot in so that the heel touches the top of the right thigh and the big toe touches the inside of the left thigh.

Push the right knee back as far as you can so as to widen the angle between the legs. The body should be stretched from the bent leg.

Now take hold of the left foot with both hands. If you can't reach the foot, hold the ankle or a cloth round the foot. Breathe in, straighten the back, and as you breathe out, pull yourself forward, aiming to lower the chest against the left thigh. Hold the position for a few moments, breathing normally. Then breathe in and sit up. Repeat on the other leg.

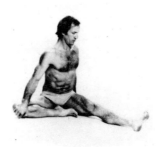

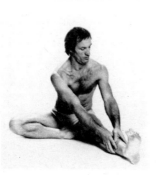

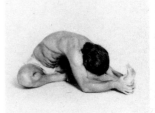

Baddha Konasana—*cobbler*

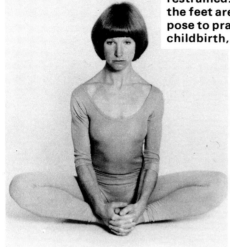

This posture is known as the cobbler pose because it is the traditional working position of Indian cobblers. Kona means angle and Baddha means caught or restrained. The angle between the legs is wide, and the feet are clasped by the hands. This is a useful pose to practise during pregnancy in preparation for childbirth, since it stretches the pelvic muscles.

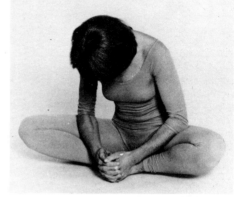

Sit in Dandasana. Bend the knees, drawing the feet towards you. Place the soles of the feet together so that the outer edges of the feet are on the floor. Clasp your hands round your toes and draw the feet in as close to the body as possible. Ideally the heels should touch the perineum. Stretch the spine so that you are sitting tall.

If your knees are on or very near the floor, press the elbows into the thighs, and as you breathe out, bend forward from the hips. You are aiming to rest your chin on the floor! Breathe in as you sit upright. Straighten and relax the legs.

Points to watch
Make sure that you are sitting well forward, not rolling back on to the base of the spine.
Use your arms to pull your back straight, but be careful not to hunch the shoulders in the process.
Try consciously to relax the muscles that are being stretched, mostly across the thighs and groin. This is the way to lower the knees, not by jerking them down.

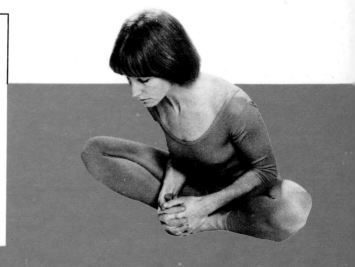

Virasana I —*hero*

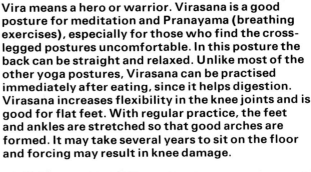

Vira means a hero or warrior. Virasana is a good posture for meditation and Pranayama (breathing exercises), especially for those who find the cross-legged postures uncomfortable. In this posture the back can be straight and relaxed. Unlike most of the other yoga postures, Virasana can be practised immediately after eating, since it helps digestion. Virasana increases flexibility in the knee joints and is good for flat feet. With regular practice, the feet and ankles are stretched so that good arches are formed. It may take several years to sit on the floor and forcing may result in knee damage.

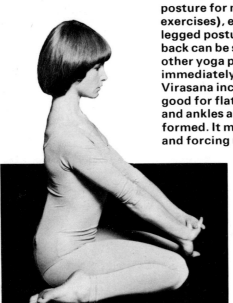

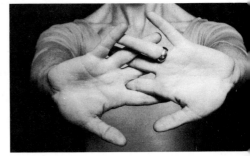

Kneel up on the floor with knees together and feet spread apart behind you, the tops of the feet resting on the floor.

Now lower yourself gently so that you sit on the floor between your feet. If your knees are stiff, put your hands on your heels and take your weight on your hands as you sit down. If you cannot sit in this position, sit on your feet as shown on the opposite page. Place your hands on your knees and sit in this position for as long as is comfortable, breathing deeply and evenly.

At first you may not be able to sit like this for more than a few seconds, but if you practise every day, your knees and ankles will become more flexible. Make sure that you are sitting comfortably for the next part of the exercise, sitting on your heels if necessary.

Interlock the fingers and stretch your arms away from you. Now straighten them above your head so that the palms are facing upwards. Stay in this position for about half a minute, breathing normally.

Relax the arms, then interlock the fingers again so that the forefinger of the other hand is nearest to you. Repeat the position with the arms stretched above your head. Drop your arms and relax them.

Now place the palms of your hands on the soles of your feet. As you breathe out, bend forward from the hips as in picture (far right). Stay in this position for up to a minute, breathing normally. Breathe in as you sit up. Then bring your feet forward and relax your legs.

The last part of the exercise (shown below right), is a more advanced variation called Supta Virasana. Only try this if you can sit easily on the floor between your feet. Hold your feet with your hands, then gently lower yourself on to your elbows. Now rest your back and then your head on the floor.

Finally, stretch your arms back on the floor behind your head. Hold this position

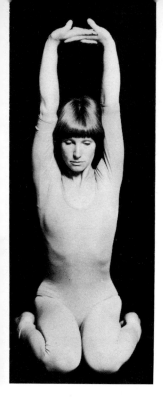

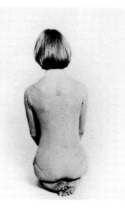
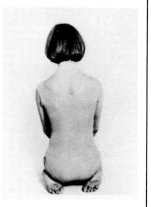
as long as you can, with deep breathing. Then hold the feet again, push up onto your elbows and sit up, on an exhalation.

Supta Virasana is a relaxing pose. It rests tired and aching legs and stretches the abdominal organs and pelvic region.

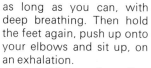

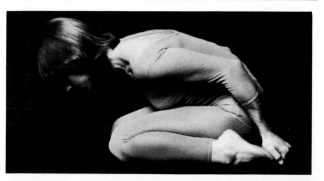

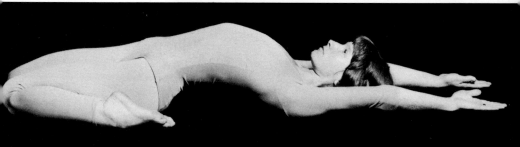

Bharadvajasana I — *twine*

This posture is the simplest of those which twist the spine. It helps to make the back supple, working on the dorsal and lumbar regions. Two more difficult twisting postures are shown later in the book. Bharadvajasana can be done even by people with very stiff backs, since the twist is a gentle one and it is not necessary to "tie the limbs in knots" to achieve it. People with arthritis may find this posture very beneficial.

Sit in Dandasana. Bend the knees, and move both legs round to the right of the body beside the hips. Sit up straight, turn the trunk to the left and bring the right arm across the body, tucking the fingers of the right hand under the outer edge of the left knee. The palm should be on the floor.

Bring the left arm behind the back, bending it at the elbow, and try to catch the right arm above the elbow with the left hand. Turn the head to look over the right shoulder. After holding the pose with normal breathing, repeat on the other side.

Points to watch
Make sure that your knees are together. If you cannot clasp the straight arm with the hand, just reach behind your back with the bent arm as far as you can.

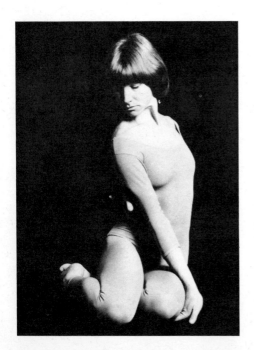
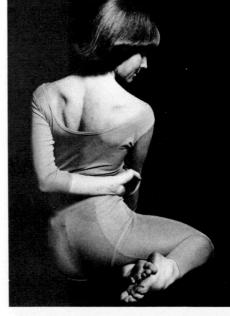

Bhujangasana—*cobra*

Bhujanga means a serpent. In this posture, from a face down position, the upper body is lifted from the floor like a snake. The spine is bent back and the chest is opened up. It is best to include at least one back bending exercise in your yoga practice, and in the cobra you can bend just as far as your back allows by taking your weight on your hands.

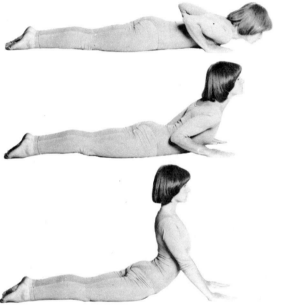

Lie on the floor face down, with your legs stretched out behind you, the tops of your feet resting on the floor. Place the palms of your hands on the floor under your shoulders, fingers pointing forwards. Rest your chin on the floor. Take a breath in and raise your head and shoulders from the floor. Take two more breaths, then gently push up with the arms to raise more of your body off the floor. When your back is flexible enough, you can straighten the arms and drop the head back. You must keep the pelvis on the ground. If the hips come off the ground, bend the arms and lower the body until they touch the floor.

Points to watch
Keep your hips on the floor.
Don't hunch your shoulders around your ears. Even in this posture, the shoulders should be dropped, with the head and neck pulled up and the chest open.

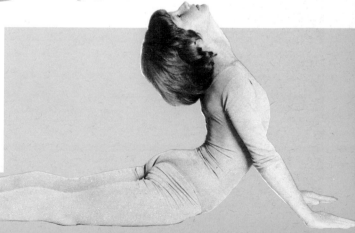

Adho Mukha Svanasana—*dog*

Adho Mukha means face down. Svana means dog. The posture resembles a dog stretching itself. This posture produces a marvellous overall stretch. It loosens the shoulders, upper back and heels, and strengthens the stomach muscles and legs. It eases tiredness in overworked legs. It also provides a good alternative posture for those who cannot do a headstand, for it has some of the same effects.

Lie face down on the floor with your legs stretched out behind, the feet up on the toes, about a foot's length apart. Place the palms of your hands on the floor under your shoulders with the fingers pointing forward. Rest your chin on the floor.

As you breathe out, push your bottom up, straighten your legs and drop your head so that you look back towards your feet. Hold this position for up to a minute, breathing normally. Then lift your head and lower your body, keeping your arms

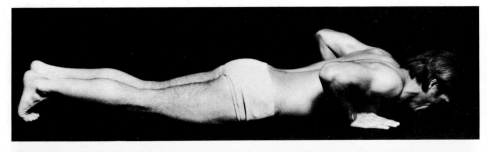

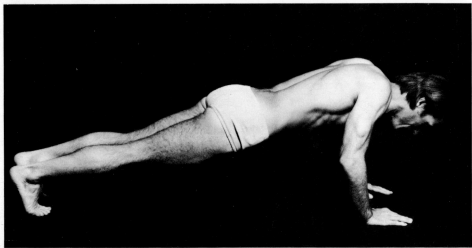

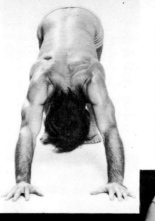

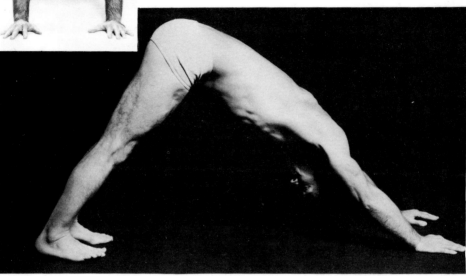

straight. The whole weight of the body should be suspended between your hands and your toes. Try not to hunch your shoulders but 'make space' between the shoulders and the ears.

Hold this position for a few seconds with normal breathing. Then, as you breathe out, push your bottom up again and drop your head down, returning to the first position. Then repeat the second position and finally rest face down on the floor and relax completely. Beginners who find this posture very hard can achieve a similar stretch in the back from a kneeling position.

Jathara Parivartanasana

Jathara means stomach or belly and Parivartana means turning around. This posture involves a twisting movement of the hips and abdomen. It strengthens the stomach muscles and is very good for all the internal abdominal organs. It also stretches the lower back and hips, bringing relief for aches in the small of the back. At first you should get another person to tether one shoulder to the ground. This is not a posture for beginners.

Lie flat on your back. Stretch the arms out sideways until they are at right angles to your body, level with the shoulders. Take a deep breath in, and as you breathe out raise both legs from the floor until they are perpendicular. Keep the thigh and knee muscles pulled tight. Now twist the hips to the right and as you breathe out, slowly lower the legs to the left, trying to bring the feet to the fingers of the left hand.

Try to keep the lower part of the back well on the floor, turning the legs from the hips.

Now drop the feet to the floor, and relax the legs. After a few seconds, as you breathe out, slowly raise the legs (keeping them straight) until they are perpendicular again. Hold this position for a few breaths, then slowly lower the legs to the floor. Relax, then repeat the movement to the other side.

Points to watch

Before you lower the legs, remember to swivel the hips in the opposite direction to that in which the legs are moving. This helps

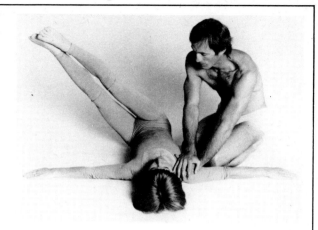

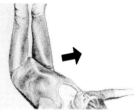

to keep the back on the floor.

If you find that the right shoulder comes off the floor when you turn the legs to the left, and vice versa, ask someone to press it down for you gently but firmly. The pressure they use should be just as much as you need, so get

them to press down only when they feel your shoulder beginning to come off the ground.

If you don't have a helper, use a heavy piece of furniture. Catch hold of this with your right hand when moving the legs to the

left, and vice versa. Beginners who find it very difficult to twist the hips with the legs in the air can do the same movement with bent knees. Start by lying on your back, knees bent and feet on the floor. Then move the hips over before raising the legs.

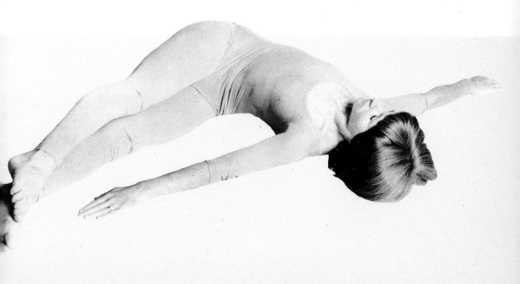

Salamba Sarvangasana—*shoulder stan*

Salamba means propped or supported. Sarvanga means the whole body (Sarva—all, Anga—limb or body). This is one of the most important yoga postures and should be included whenever possible in your yoga practice. B.K.S. Iyengar calls Sarvangasana the "Mother of asanas" as it benefits the entire body. Some of its effects are: healthy functioning of the thyroid and parathyroid glands; soothing of the nerves and relief from constipation and headaches.

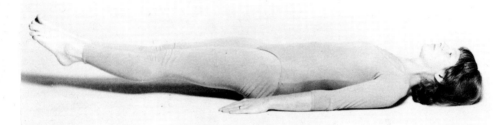

Lie flat on your back on the floor. Make sure that you have a substantial rug, blanket or carpet underneath you, and that your head, neck, shoulders and upper arms are all on the rug. This is to protect your neck. If your neck is stiff then move the head onto the floor. See that your head is quite straight, in line with your body.

Method for beginners
Instead of bringing the legs up straight, bend the knees and draw them towards your chest. As you breathe out, lift the hips from the floor and prop them on your hands. Push up with the hands until all the trunk is off the floor, then finally straighten the legs. Don't let the body sink down, but stretch up with the trunk and legs.

Take a few deep breaths, then on an exhalation slowly raise both legs until they are perpendicular. Take a breath in, and as you breathe out, raise the legs further and lift the hips and back from the floor, pressing down with the palms of your hands to help you lift.

When most of the upper body is off the floor, bend the arms and support the back on your hands. Now straighten your legs. Pull up with the entire body to raise as much of it as possible off the floor, at the same time pushing it up with the supporting hands.

Eventually only the back of the head, the neck, the shoulders and the upper arms rest on the floor, and

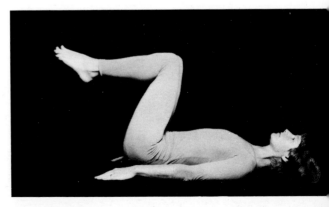

58

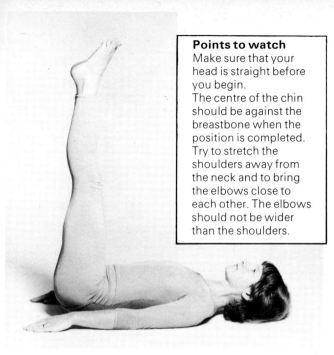

Points to watch
Make sure that your head is straight before you begin.
The centre of the chin should be against the breastbone when the position is completed. Try to stretch the shoulders away from the neck and to bring the elbows close to each other. The elbows should not be wider than the shoulders.

the breastbone presses against the chin to form a chinlock. The head should not move throughout the exercise. Make sure your body is in a straight line. You may need someone to tell you whether your legs are straight.

To straighten the legs, tighten the thigh muscles and stretch up vertically. At first, breathing will feel strange, in fact the whole position will feel odd, but you soon become accustomed to it. Try to increase the time you stay in shoulder stand to five minutes or more.

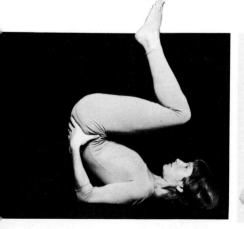

Halasana—*plough*

Halasana is a continuation of Sarvangasana, the shoulder stand, and has similar beneficial effects. In addition, the abdominal organs are "toned up" through being contracted, as in Paschimottanasana, the forward bend. Halasana helps to relieve backache and eases stiffness in the back, shoulders and elbows. Practising Halasana also brings improvement in Paschimottanasana. People with high blood pressure are advised to do Halasana with feet on a chair before attempting the shoulder stand.

First of all, do the shoulder stand. Then slowly lower the legs towards the floor, keeping them quite straight. Take them as far over as you can without bending the knees. When the feet are on the floor, tighten the knees and stretch the back of the legs. Straighten the back by pulling the hips up vertically. Rest in this position, breathing normally, for one to five minutes. As in the shoulder stand, breathing will feel strange at first, but there should be no strain.

When you have a steady position, stretch your arms back so that your hands reach towards your feet. Try walking your feet away from your head and also pulling the spine up straight.

Now stretch the arms behind your back. Clasp your hands by interlocking the fingers, turn the palms inwards so that the little fingers rest on the floor and straighten the elbows. This position gives an extra stretch to the spine.

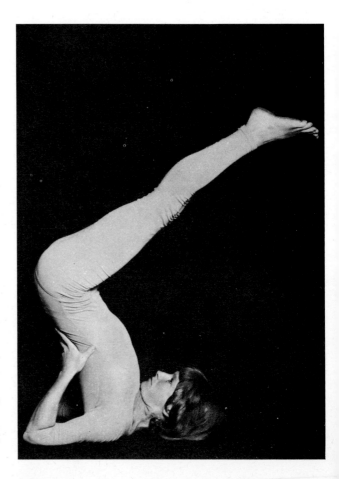

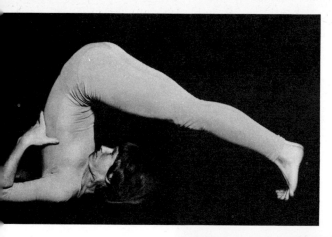

Points to watch
As in all the inverted postures, the body should not be allowed to sag or "just hang there". It should be taut and stretched. So make sure that the legs are straight and well stretched, and the back pulled up. You should aim to make the back vertical, not rounded.

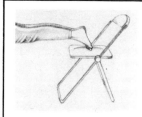

If you cannot reach the floor with your toes, place a chair or similar object behind you and rest your feet on that.

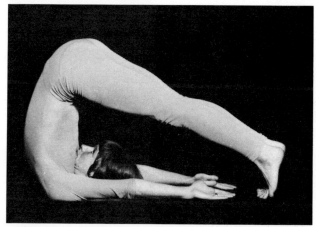

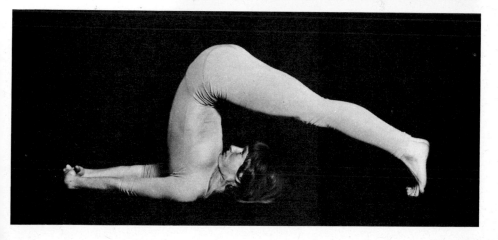

Karnapidasana

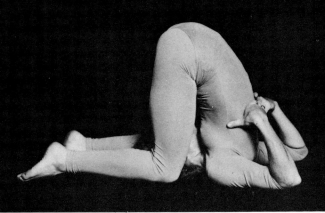

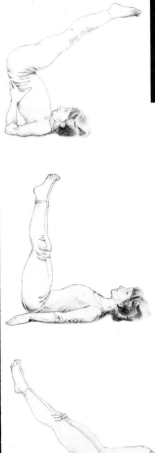

Karna means ear and Pida means pressure. After Halasana has become easy bend the knees and place them each side of the head, pressing against the ears.

The knees and the top of the feet should be resting on the floor. Either keep the hands on the back or clasp the fingers and stretch the arms behind the back as in Halasana. Stay in this position for up to a minute with normal breathing. Then straighten the legs and return to the shoulder stand, supporting the hips with the hands.

This position is a very restful one. Although the spine is being stretched, it is a passive stretch, the force of gravity pulling the legs down, and the trunk, heart and legs are rested. It is a soothing and comforting position to hold, for one feels withdrawn, enclosed and self-contained.

To come down from the shoulder stand, keep the legs straight and drop the hips down and away from the head, so that the back and legs are at an angle.

Now lower the hips and back to the floor so that the legs are perpendicular.

Slowly lower the legs to the floor.

Beginners: bend the knees while in the shoulder stand, then gently roll the back onto the floor.

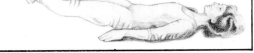

Savasana—*corpse*

This is perhaps the most important posture in the book. It is not as easy as it looks. Its purpose is to relax the body completely and to keep the mind still. One should end every yoga practice with Savasana: it removes fatigue caused by doing the other postures and calms the mind, so that one finishes the practice feeling refreshed and invigorated. The physical stretching and mental concentration involved in the other postures prepare the body and mind for relaxation in Savasana.

Lie flat on your back on the floor making sure that you are warm and comfortable. Flex your feet up, stretching the heels, then relax them so that they flop out sideways. Push the shoulders down.

Place the arms a little way from the body, the hands relaxed with palms uppermost. Settle the back comfortably on the floor and check that your head is straight. Now be aware of every part of the body, from toes to scalp, and consciously relax it. Pay special attention to the face, eyes, jaw, tongue and throat. If the mind wanders, bring it back to the sound of your breathing which should become fine and slow.

Points to watch
Lay your head carefully on the floor so that it rests on the centre back, slightly stretching the back of the neck, so the chin is down.
Check that no muscle is tensed.
Stay in this pose for at least five minutes, enjoying inner calm and stillness.

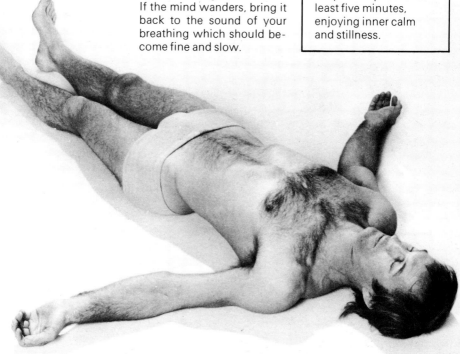

Surya Namaskars—*salute to the sun*

This is an ancient Indian exercise which combines six yoga postures in a sequence of ten movements. Four of the positions are repeated. The original Sanskrit name of the exercise, Sashtanga Surya Namaskar, means obeisance to the sun with eight points of the body. The eight points are the parts of the body which touch the ground in the fifth position: two toes, two knees, chest, forehead and two palms. The best time to do this exercise is in the morning. It stretches and tones the whole body, so is an effective way of waking up. It can be repeated as many times as you like, though it is best to start gradually.

1. Stand with feet together, knees straight, back stretched up but not tense. Join the palms of the hands in front of the chest and breathe in slowly and deeply. Breathe out as you move into the second position.

2. Bend forward from the hips until the hands are on the ground in front of you on either side of your legs. Keep your legs quite straight. Try to bring your nose and forehead to your knees, and keep your chin tucked in against your chest. Pull the stomach in. Then breathe in while you move into the third position.

3. Keeping your hands and arms in the same place, stretch one foot as far as you can behind you, at the same time lifting up your head and trying to bend back. Now breathe out as you move to the fourth position.

4. This is the same as the dog pose on page 55. Take the second foot back and straighten both legs. Try to press your heels flat onto the

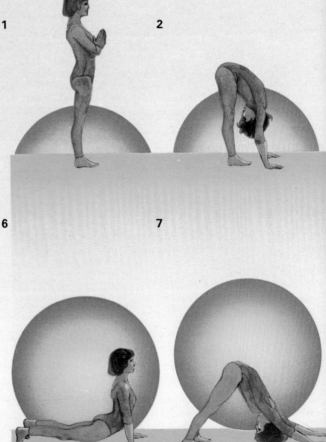

ground. Drop your head down so that your chin is tucked into your chest again. Keep your arms straight and try to flatten and extend the spine. Take another breath in and breathe out as you go into the fifth position.

5. Keeping hands and feet where they are, bend your arms and lower your body to the ground, touching the ground only with your toes, knees, chest and forehead. Pull your stomach in as you breathe out.

6. As you breathe in, lift your head and bend backwards, straightening the arms and legs so that the weight of the whole body is on hands and toes.

7. As you breathe out, lift your bottom into the air, drop your head with chin tucked into chest and straighten your legs. This is the same as position four.

8. As you breathe in, bring one leg forward so the foot rests between the hands.

Look up and bend back as in position three. Breathe out fully as you move into the ninth position.

9. This is a repeat of position two. Bring the other foot forward next to the first. Straighten your legs and tuck your chin in.

10. Breathe in as you lift your hands off the ground and stand up with a straight back, unbending at the hips. Join the palms in front of the chest.

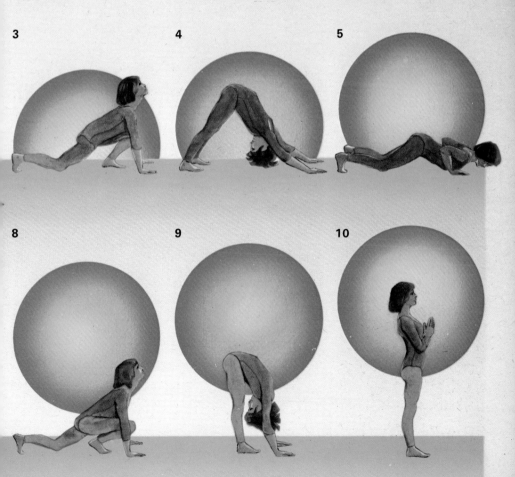

Parivrtta Trikonasana—*reverse triangle*

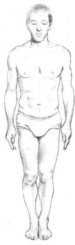

Parivrtta means revolved and Trikona a triangle. This is a counter-pose to Uttihita Trikonasana, shown on page 36. You will feel a strong pull on the hamstrings and thighs and a stretch in the hips and lower back as the hips turn, and you will feel the chest expanding as you twist the body further round to the back. Like Uttihita Trikonasana and the tree posture, this pose should be done against a wall at first, as there may be a tendency to overbalance.

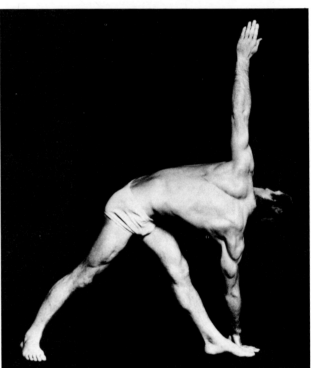

Stand in Tadasana. Place the feet 1 metre apart, turning the right foot 90 degrees and the left foot about 60 degrees to the right. Breathe in and raise the arms to shoulder level. As you breathe out, turn the hips, swing the upper body round and drop the left hand down towards the right foot. Stretch the right arm up and turn the head to look at the right thumb. Hold this pose for up to half a minute breathing normally, then breathe in as you straighten up. Repeat on the left.

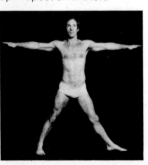

Points to watch
Keep both legs straight with the knees pulled tight.
Keep the outer edge of the back foot well on the floor.
If you can't reach your foot with the lower hand, hold the leg as low as possible without bending the knees. Stretch your arms and your back across the shoulders.

Padangusthasana—*toe catch*

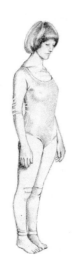

Pada means foot and Angustha means the big toe. Padangusthasana involves bending from the hips, and catching hold of the big toes. If you cannot reach your toes, hold your legs as low as you can, without bending your knees. This posture tones the abdominal organs and stretches the spine in the lower back. This can be beneficial for people with slipped discs, but in these circumstances it should only be attempted under the guidance of an expert teacher.

Stand in Tadasana. Place the feet about a foot apart. As you breathe out, bend forward and catch the big toes with the first two fingers, keeping the knees pulled tight. Grasp the toes firmly and look upwards, raising the head and trying to hollow the back.

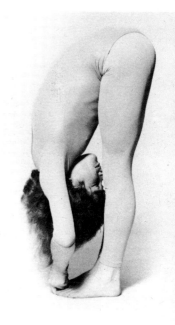

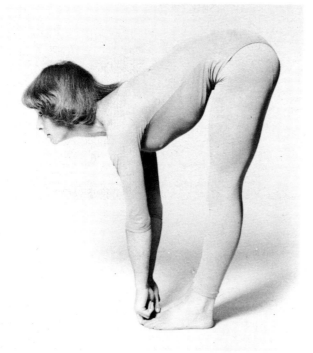

Take one or two breaths, then exhale and pull the chest down towards the knees, using the grip on the toes to pull you forward. Hold this position for a few seconds, breathing normally, then inhale and raise the head again, stretching the back (left). Release the toes and stand up, returning to Tadasana.

Upavistha Konasana

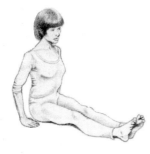

Upavistha means seated and Kona means angle. This posture consists of a forward bend with the legs at a wide angle. It stretches the hamstrings and stimulates the pelvic region. At first you may not be able to spread the legs very wide, or to bend very far forward. Don't force yourself into position—just go as far as you can. The important thing is to keep the legs straight and to bend forward from the hips, even if the movement is very slight. Don't bring your head to the floor by humping the back. If you wish to extend further forward when already in position, do so on an out breath.

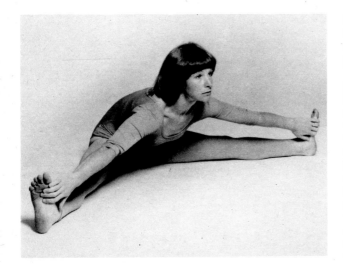

Sit in Dandasana, with legs stretched out in front. Separate the legs as wide apart as possible with straight knees. Try to sit up straight by pushing with hands on the floor behind you. If this is easy, try to catch hold of your toes or clasp your feet with your hands. Straighten the back, extending the ribs forward. Take two or three deep breaths, then, as you breathe out, bend forward as if to put the chest on the floor. Stay in this position for a few moments with normal breathing. Then inhale as you sit up. Relax the legs.

Points to watch
Keep the legs very straight, the entire backs of the legs on the floor.
Sit well forward with a straight back before bending forward.
Don't allow yourself to sink backwards on to the base of the spine.
Remember to breathe normally while holding the posture.

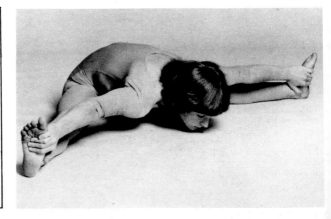

Prasarita Padottanasana

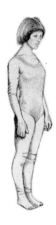

Prasarita means spread wide and Pada means foot. This posture stretches the legs, especially the hamstrings, the ankles and the groin. It also pulls up the arches of the feet. When the head touches the floor, the blood runs freely to the chest and the head, so this is a good posture for those who cannot do Sirsasana, the headstand. Before bending forward, stand for a few moments with the feet spread wide and the hands on the hips, pulling the spine up straight. If this is very uncomfortable, don't proceed with the rest of the pose, but simply practise this first stage until the legs are stretched wide enough to put your hands on the floor.

Stand in Tadasana. Spread the legs wide apart, 1¾ metres, and place the hands on the hips. Pull the knees up tight, exhale and bend forward, placing the hands on the floor. Breathe in and raise the head, trying to hollow the back. As you breathe out, bend the elbows and bring the head down towards the floor. Keep your weight on the feet. Stay like this for up to half a minute, breathing normally. Inhale

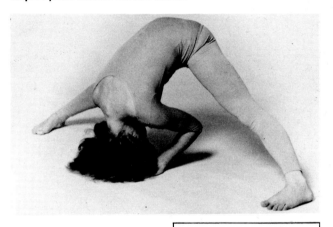

and straighten your arms, raising your head and hollowing the back. Then wriggle the feet in towards each other and stand up.

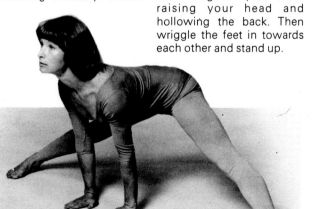

Points to watch
Make sure that the feet are parallel, with the weight mostly on the outer edge of the feet and the arches pulled up. Dig the big toe into the floor. Keep the knees pulled up tight throughout.
When the elbows bend, bend them back between the legs, not out sideways.
The feet, hands and head should eventually be in line.

Marichyasana III

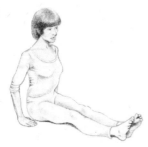

This is one of a group of postures named after the sage Marichi, son of Brahma and grandfather of Surya, the Sun God. Like Bharadvajasana, it twists the spine, but the twist is more intense. This is a very good posture for backache and lumbago and it loosens the shoulder joints. It is especially recommended for people with excess fat around the waist.

Sit in Dandasana. Bend the left knee and place the left foot flat on the floor, so that the shin is vertical, the calf folded against the thigh.

The left heel should be pulled in close to the body, with the inside edge of the foot against the right thigh. As you breathe out, turn the body to the left about 90 degrees and place the right elbow outside the left knee.

Move the right shoulder beyond the left knee and extend the right arm so that the body is twisted further to the left. Take another breath in, and as you breathe out bend the right elbow and reach the right hand behind the waist.

Breathe in and as you exhale bring the left arm behind the back and try to clasp the hands. When you can hold the hands, you can use the grip to pull the body still more to the left. Turn the head to look over the left shoulder.

Hold this position breathing normally, then return to Dandasana. Repeat the position on the other side.

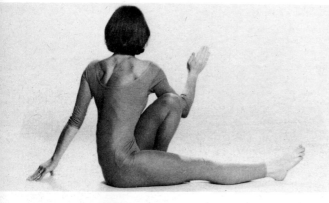

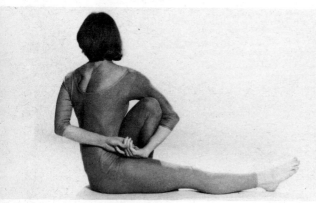

Points to watch
The spine should be stretched up.
There should be no downward pressure on the abdomen.
If you cannot join hands then stop in first pose looking over the left shoulder.

Paripurna Navasana—*boat*

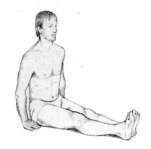

Nava means boat or ship. Paripurna means complete. This posture is said to resemble a boat with oars. It strengthens the back and the stomach muscles. You can feel the effect on the latter if you hold the position for only a few seconds! B.K.S. Iyengar says of this posture and its companion pose, Ardha Navasana: "The two asanas bring life and vigour to the back and enable us to grow old gracefully and comfortably."

Sit in Dandasana, with your legs stretched out in front. As you breathe out, tip the body backwards slightly, raising the legs from the floor. Keep the legs very stiff. Take the hands from the floor and stretch the arms straight out in front of you, palms facing each other. The arms should be on a level with the shoulders, parallel to the floor.

The back should be kept straight. Ideally, no part of the spine should touch the floor, the weight balancing on the buttocks. At first you will probably topple backwards, as you try to balance. When you can balance, work to pull the back up from the floor. Gradually increase the time you stay in this pose to one minute. Don't hold it too long to begin with.

Points to watch
Do not hold your breath while holding the pose, try to breathe lightly, if anything pausing after the out breath.

If you find it very difficult to raise the legs from Dandasana start with bent knees and the toes just off the floor, straightening the legs from there.

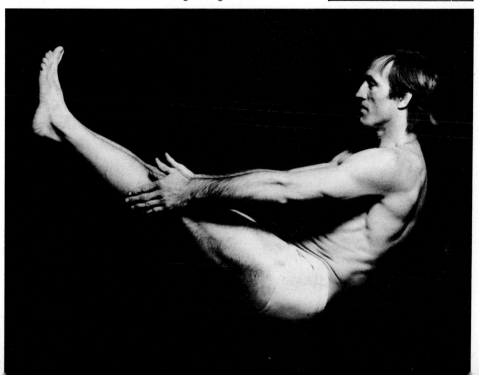

Ardha Matsyendrasana I

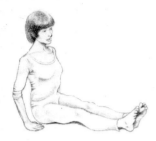

This posture is named after Matsyendra, Lord of the Fishes, a god who is associated with the study and practice of yoga. Ardha means half, and this posture is an easier form of an intense spinal twist. The benefits are similar to those of Marichyasana III on page 70, but somewhat intensified since there is a greater degree of movement. Nonetheless, some people may find it easier to lock themselves into this position than Marichyasana 111.

Sit in Dandasana, with the legs stretched out in front. Bend the left knee and draw the foot in to the body.

Sit on the foot so that the left heel is under the left buttock. The outer edge of the foot and the little toe should be on the ground.

Then bend the right knee

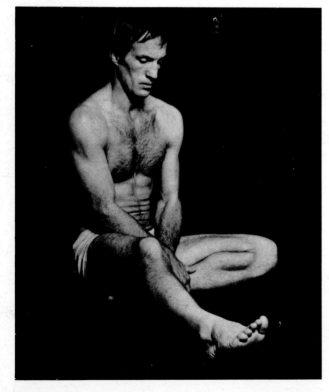

and move the right leg across and over the left thigh; place the right foot on the floor outside the left thigh, with the outer edge of the right ankle touching the thigh. Now turn the trunk to the right and place the left armpit over the right knee. As you breathe out, straighten the left arm and bring it across the body in front of the right knee, placing the left hand on the right foot.

Take a breath in, and as you breathe out bend the right arm and take the right hand behind the back. Turn the head so that you look over the right shoulder. Hold the position for up to a minute with normal breathing.

Then release the hands and straighten first the right and then the left leg. Now repeat the pose on the other side, holding it for the same length of time. If you find it difficult to sit on the foot, then sit on the floor and bring the foot in close to the body.

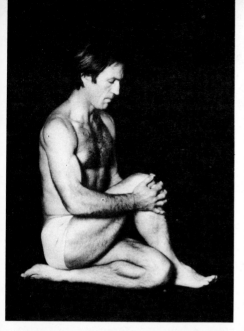

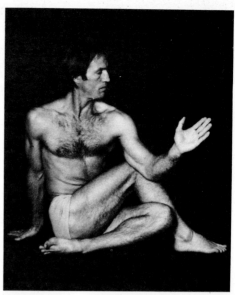

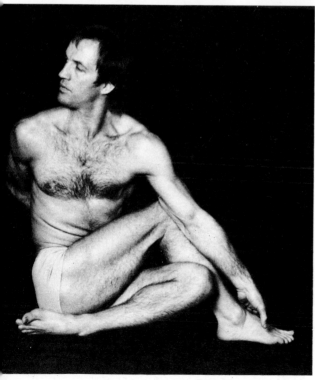

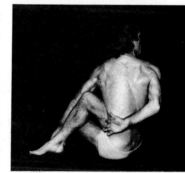

Points to watch
Make sure that the out-
stretched arm locks the
bent knee tightly, so
that there is no space
between the armpit and
the bent knee.
Keep the back as
straight as possible, so
that the spine is
stretched up while it is
being twisted sideways.
This pose is not suitable
for beginners.

Ustrasana—*camel*

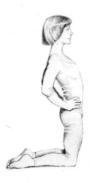

This posture opens out the chest, correcting drooping shoulders and hunched backs. It gives the spine a good backward stretch and can be practised even by very elderly people, although for some people (of all ages) it may be difficult at first to achieve the complete posture.

To obtain maximum stretch on the spine, it is important to bend back from the waist, keeping the thighs and hips vertical. Do not let the body slant backwards from the knees, but keep the hips pushed forwards. This is a good counter-balancing pose to the forward bends such as Paschimottanasana.

Kneel up on the floor, keeping the knees, legs and feet 30 cms apart. Place the hands on the hips and stretch the spine up and slightly back, opening the chest.

Take a breath in, and as you exhale drop your arms back and place your hands over your heels. The arms should be turned outwards. If you can, rest the palms of your hands along the soles of your feet. Pressing against the feet with the hands, drop your head back and push the hips forward so that the spine is stretched backwards. Hold this position up to half a minute, breathing normally.

Beginners should try at first with the toes tucked in underneath the feet so that the heels are lifted slightly off the floor.

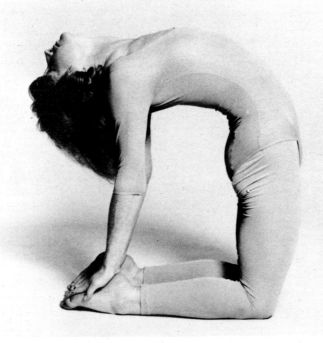

Salabhasana—*locust*

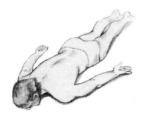

This posture is a good exercise for the hips, abdomen, pelvis and lower back. The spine becomes more supple and pain in the lower back can be eased. The position requires considerable muscular effort, and there is a tendency to hold the breath while holding the pose. Try to breathe normally.

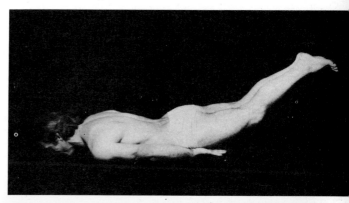

Lie flat on the floor face downwards, tops of the feet resting on the floor and arms by the sides. The legs should be together. Rest your chin on the floor. Take a breath in, and as you breathe out, raise the legs from the floor as high as you can while keeping them straight.

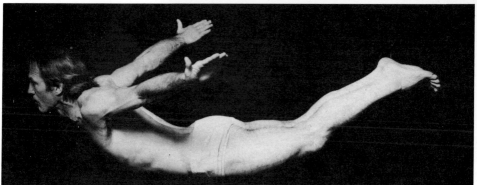

Contract the buttocks and the thigh muscles, and try to keep the legs together. Breathe normally while you hold the position as long as you can. Lower the legs and relax.

Now repeat the exercise, raising the head, chest and arms as well as the legs.

Lift the ribs from the floor and stretch the arms out behind you. Only the stomach should be resting on the floor. Again, remember to keep the legs straight and together. Hold the position as long as you can with normal breathing, then lie flat on the floor and relax.

Points to watch
If you find it very difficult to raise your legs in the first position, try tucking your fists underneath your thighs before lifting up.

Urdhva Dhanurasana—*wheel*

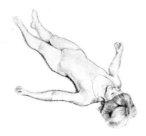

This posture is sometimes called Chakrasana—Chakra means wheel. Urdhva means upwards and Dhanu means a bow, so this could also be called the bow posture. It can only be done by people with a strong back and supple spine. It stretches the spine fully, strengthens the arms and wrists and has a soothing effect, like all the inverted poses.

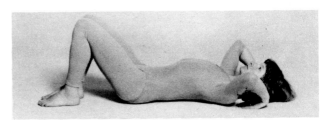

Lie flat on your back on the floor. Bend your elbows and place your hands under your shoulders, palms on the floor and fingers pointing towards your feet. Bend the knees and bring your feet in towards your hips.

Breathe in, and as you breathe out, push up on your hands and feet, straightening the arms and lifting your body from the floor so that your back forms an arch. Hold this position for about half a minute, breathing normally. Then breathe out as you lower the body to the floor and relax.

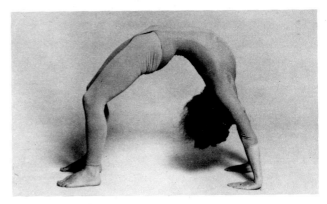

When you can hold the wheel comfortably, try the variation shown in the bottom picture. After lifting your back and straightening the arms, straighten your legs, keeping the feet together. This bends the spine further. Hold for a few moments with normal breathing, then bend your knees and relax on the floor. This pose is not suitable for beginners.

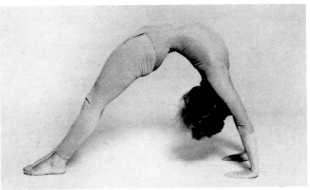

Anantasana

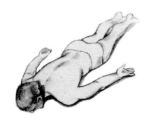

Ananta is the name of Visnu and also of the thousand-headed serpent on which Visnu sleeps, according to Hindu mythology. Ananta means literally "without end", and the serpent is a symbol of eternity. This posture is a good exercise for the pelvis and it stretches the hamstring muscles, as you will feel when you do it.

Begin by lying flat on the floor. As you breathe out, roll onto your right side. Prop your head on your right hand. Bend your left knee and catch hold of your big toe.

As you breathe out, straighten the arm and leg together so that they are stretched up vertically. Hold the position for a few moments with normal breathing, then exhale as you replace the arm and leg. Roll onto the back, turn onto the left side and repeat. Then relax.

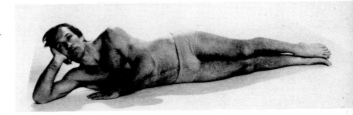

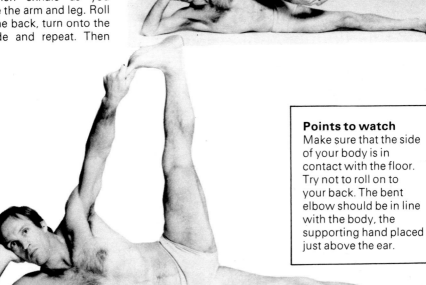

Points to watch
Make sure that the side of your body is in contact with the floor. Try not to roll on to your back. The bent elbow should be in line with the body, the supporting hand placed just above the ear.

Sirsasana—*headstand*

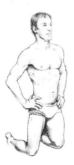

Sirsasana is traditionally known as the king of the Asanas. As in Sarvangasana, the upside-down position benefits the entire body : the force of gravity pulling in the opposite direction from usual has a rejuvenating effect. Since in the headstand there is no chinlock, the blood flows freely to the brain, relieving mental fatigue, and to the pineal and pituitary glands which control the body's growth and health. The beginner in yoga is advised to master Sarvangasana and the standing postures before attempting headstand. Once you do start to practise Sirsasana, it should be performed before the other postures, while the body is still fresh.

Kneel on the floor near your blanket which should be folded several times to make it thick. Interlock the fingers firmly. Rest the crown of the head on the blanket, the back of the head against the cupped hands, straighten the legs, walk the toes towards the head and on an out breath lift both legs together so that you are balanced as in middle picture. Slowly straighten the legs, and stretch them. Hold as long as you can, then bend the knees and slowly bring the legs down.

Make sure that the elbows are not wider apart than the shoulders.

The weight of the body should be on the crown of the head alone. The body should be straight—back of head, trunk, back of thighs and heels all in line. The waist and hips should not be pushed forward. Stretch the legs fully, especially the backs.

The beginner is advised to get help from a teacher or friend, or use a wall (10 cms away, preferably a corner) for support. The body should be as in Tadasana page 35, but the other way up.

Padmasana—*lotus*

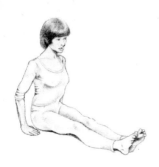

The lotus posture is the classic yoga posture for meditation. It locks the legs in position, so there is no danger of falling over and no muscular effort needed to hold them there. It keeps the back very straight. All this is conducive to an alert relaxed mind. Once the knees and ankles are supple enough, the lotus is a relaxing pose, and can be held comfortably for quite a long time. The Hatha Yoga Pradipika describes how to assume lotus with beautiful simplicity: 'Place each foot on the opposite thigh.' It may take several years of practice to achieve this. If you cannot, then start with Ardha Padmasana as pictured on page 81.

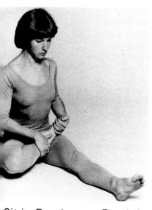

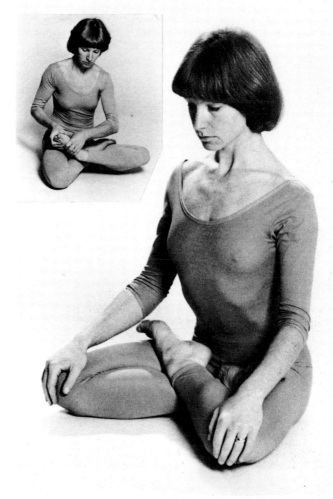

Sit in Dandasana. Bend the right knee, pick up the right foot and place it on the opposite thigh so that the heel is near the navel. Now bend the left knee, pick up the left foot and place it over the right thigh in the same position. The soles of the feet should be turned up.

Straighten the spine from the base to the back of the neck. Either place the hands on the knees, or place them palms up, one on top of the other, where the feet cross.

Change the leg position, so that the right foot comes over the left.

Pranayama—*breathing*

Pranayama is control of the breathing and is the fourth of the classical eight limbs of yoga. Breathing is of great importance in yoga, not only because it keeps the body alive by supplying it with oxygen, but also because the act of breathing is believed to draw vital force into the organism. This force or Prana is described as the life force or cosmic energy, and has been interpreted as psychic energy.

Prana means breath or life force, and Ayama means pause. Pranayama exercises consist of combinations of breathing techniques, including alternate nostril breathing and prolonged breath holding. Untrained practice of Pranayama can damage the heart, lungs and nervous system. There is a close link between breathing and psychological states (compare your breathing when calm or nearly asleep with the way you breathe when nervous or excited). Yogis regard breathing as the bridge between body and mind, and between the conscious and the subconscious.

Beginners in yoga should learn to improve their normal breathing before studying Pranayama. Many people do not use their lungs fully, so their breathing is shallow and rapid. This means that the body tissues are deprived of oxygen, the lungs cannot get rid of all the waste matter produced during respiration, and even the kidneys and bowels work less efficiently, since in deep breathing the movement of the diaphragm stimulates

them. The whole system becomes sluggish and the heart is under strain.

Ujjayi
This is a preparatory exercise which can be done even when walking about once you are familiar with it. It is a slow, rhythmical breath which expands the ribcage and lungs, soothes the nerves and tones the system. First of all, sit or lie on the floor with a straight back. Start with a deep exhalation, then expand the chest to draw in the air. Don't contract the nostrils, which should be relaxed, but slightly contract the back of the nose, feeling the passage of air against it. This makes a sound like a faint snore.

Continue to breathe in and out rhythmically, being aware of the movement of the upper ribs, chest and stomach, which contract as you breathe out and expand as you breathe in. When breathing out, pull the stomach muscles in firmly to expel as much air as possible.

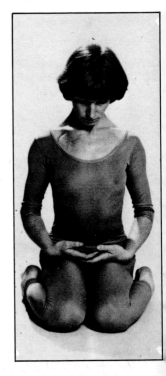

▶ A simple posture for practising deep breathing, Virasana, the kneeling pose which is also suitable for meditation.

Meditation

The Eastern religious philosophies such as Vedanta and Buddhism are based on the experience of meditation. The practice of meditation is found in all the major religions including Christianity, on the assumption that Truth is to be found within our own consciousness and not elsewhere. By exploring the mind we become conscious of an area of ourselves beyond the ordinary mind; hence the term transcendental meditation.

The interpretations of the meditation experience vary. The Hindu Vedanta talks of realizing the Self which is the universal Spirit in all things (Brahman). Buddhism describes it as the realization of 'no-self'. But both recognize the experience in which the sense of ego disappears, so that the person or seer becomes one with the seen, and there is a total lack of self-consciousness in the literal sense of the word. This experience is generally referred to as Samadhi, and is the third of the traditional stages in yoga meditation. The two previous stages are

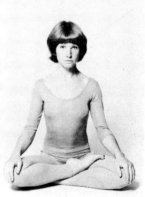

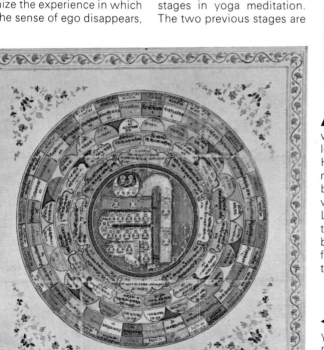

▲ There are several variations of the cross-legged seat. This is the Half Lotus and is a classic meditation posture. It can be comfortable for those who cannot sit in full Lotus. Place one foot on the ground close to the body, and place the other foot on the opposite thigh or just in front.

◄ Symbolic pictures or yantras, like this one representing the sacred symbol Om, are a traditional aid for yoga meditation.

Dharana, concentration on one subject, and Dhyana, contemplation. The Yoga Sutras describe Dharana as "attention fixed upon an object", Dhyana as "union of mind and object", and Samadhi as "Illumination, where union as union disappears, only the meaning of the object on which the attention is fixed being present".

In Samadhi, the mind is cleared of all distracting thoughts so that it reflects like a mirror whatever it is directed towards, whether an object or one's inner self. It has been described as a lake on which the waves and ripples gradually subside, until the surface is smooth enough to give a clear reflection.

The process of stilling the waves is what takes place during meditation; indeed it may begin during the practice of the yoga postures and relaxation. The ability to "empty" the mind in this way can be carried into everyday life, so that one can see things as they are, undistorted by one's own prejudices.

There are innumerable techniques for clearing the mind, and each person has to find that which suits him best. Some of these are: concentration on an object or picture, real or imagined; concentration on a quotation; repetition of sounds (Mantras) aloud or inwardly; and concentration on the sound of one's breathing (this is a kind of Mantra).

One of the best exercises for the beginner to practise is a technique of self-awareness, in which one lets the mind wander in its usual fashion, but instead of drifting along with it, one observes what the mind is doing. The mind naturally follows trains of thought linked by associations often produced by sense impressions. It remembers past incidents and plans the future. When practising this exercise, try not to be drawn by these thoughts, just watch

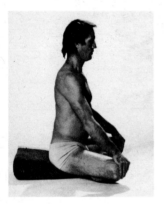

▲ A cushion under the buttocks can relieve pressure on the knees and ankles and help you to sit with a straight back.

▶ Even Indian yogis may have difficulty in sitting comfortably with crossed legs. This seventeenth century statue shows a yogi using a band to take the strain.

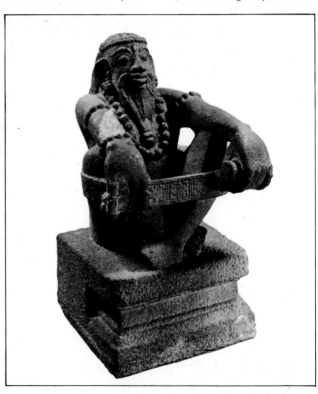

them arise and disappear. If you do start to drift with them, bring yourself back to the present by observing what is happening in the mind and body right now. No thoughts should be suppressed, even if they alarm you by floating up from the subconscious unexpectedly. Just watch them and don't identify yourself with them.

This technique is a valuable aid to concentration and meditation. It can be practised as a form of 'active' meditation during any ordinary activity, by just bringing the mind back to whatever one is actually doing.

Posture

It is very important to have a comfortable posture if you are to sit quite still for half an hour or so and forget about your body. This does not mean that you have to sit in lotus posture, but that the back and back of the neck must be straight and in line, either self-supported or supported by a chair back or even the floor. The chin should be tucked in so that the ears are in line with the shoulders. Lying on the floor is a good position, but there is a danger of falling sleep.

The symmetrical sitting postures such as the lotus require least effort to maintain, but for people who have lost the natural ability to sit like this it takes a lot of practice to achieve a comfortable cross-legged position. The lotus is ideal for meditation because the legs are locked in position, form-ing a firm base for a straight back. However, if it is excruciatingly uncomfortable, its purpose is defeated. Alternative cross-legged postures can be used, or a kneeling posture, or perhaps best for some people is a straight-backed chair.

The hands should be relaxed, placed either on the knees or thighs, or cupped one inside the other near the navel. The chin is tucked in and the eyes are lowered to look at the floor about a metre ahead of the body.

Practice

It is very important to establish a habit of posture, and also of place and time. Choose a quiet, pleasant room and practise at the same time each day, either morning or evening. Have a special rug, cushion or chair. Wear loose, comfortable clothes, and keep warm. Don't be in a hurry—leave all that behind you when you sit down. And don't expect anything. Try not to conceptualize the experience beforehand. Think of the exercise at first as a pleasant antidote to life's hustle and bustle. You are deliberately taking time out. When you have learnt skill in doing this the experience and benefits will happen of their own accord.

To begin with, do as much as you can, using whatever technique suits you best. For example, start with some deep breathing. Then consciously assume a mental attitude of love and harmony towards everyone. Sit quietly for a while watching the mind and being aware of the present moment. Then begin concentration on an object that has good associations, or on the rhythm of your own breathing. Gradually increase the time you spend sitting. Practise regularly, but don't strain. Concentration is relaxation.

You can use an incense stick or taper to time yourself. A candle flame is found by many people to be a good object for concentration. Watch it steadily without straining the eyes. You can try shutting your eyes and retaining the image of the flame for as long as you can.

"With upright body, head, and neck, which rest still and move not; with inner gaze which is not restless, but rests still between the eyebrows . . . let the seeker quietly lead the mind into the Spirit, and let all his thoughts be silence.

"And whenever the mind unsteady and restless strays away from the Spirit, let him ever and for ever lead it again to the Spirit...

"Then his soul is a lamp whose light is steady, for it burns in a shelter where no winds come." Bhagavadgita.

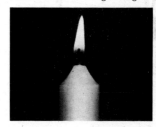

Planning a programme

This page shows a progressive programme for beginners: start with the left hand column for a week or so, then progress from one colour to the next, The opposite page shows a selection of postures for each day of the week, for more advanced students.

	Week	1	2	3	4	5
	Tadasana – mountain					
	Uttihita Trikonasana – triangle					
	Uttihita Parsvakonasana					
	Virabhadrasana I – warrior					
	Virabhadrasana II					
	Uttanasana – relaxed					
	Vrksasana – tree					
	Parsvottanasana					
	Dandasana – staff					
	Paschimottanasana – forward bend					

	Week	1	2	3	4	5
	Janu Sirsasana					
	Baddha Konasana – cobbler					
	Virasana I – hero					
	Bharadvajasana I – twine					
	Bhujangasana – cobra					
	Adho Mukha Svanasana – dog					
	Jathara Parivartanasana					
	Salamba Sarvangasana – shoulder stand					
	Halasana – plough					
	Savasana – corpse					

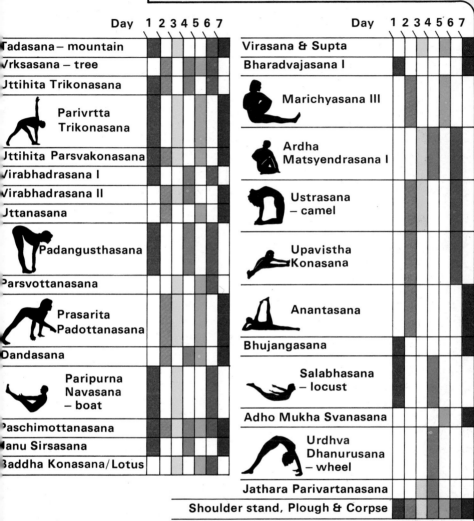

Day 1 2 3 4 5 6 7

Left column poses:
- Tadasana – mountain
- Vrksasana – tree
- Uttihita Trikonasana
- Parivrtta Trikonasana
- Uttihita Parsvakonasana
- Virabhadrasana I
- Virabhadrasana II
- Uttanasana
- Padangusthasana
- Parsvottanasana
- Prasarita Padottanasana
- Dandasana
- Paripurna Navasana – boat
- Paschimottanasana
- Janu Sirsasana
- Baddha Konasana/Lotus

Day 1 2 3 4 5 6 7

Right column poses:
- Virasana & Supta
- Bharadvajasana I
- Marichyasana III
- Ardha Matsyendrasana I
- Ustrasana – camel
- Upavistha Konasana
- Anantasana
- Bhujangasana
- Salabhasana – locust
- Adho Mukha Svanasana
- Urdhva Dhanurusana – wheel
- Jathara Parivartanasana
- Shoulder stand, Plough & Corpse

The above is simply a guide for use until you have established the form of practice which suits you best. Try to include Shoulder Stand and Forward Bend whenever possible, and always finish with relaxation in the Corpse pose. The routine can be split, so that Shoulder Stand, Plough and Corpse are done in the evening and the rest earlier in the day. Or do the standing postures in the morning and the rest in the evening. If you can do Headstand, include it before Shoulder Stand. If you have really little time for a yoga routine, try the following:
Morning: Salute to the Sun (page 64-5).
Evening: Dog pose or Cobra, Forward Bend, Shoulder Stand, Plough and Corpse.

List of postures

This list of additional postures is for reference only. There are hundreds of yoga Asanas; the number has grown through the centuries, for Hatha yoga is an experimental science. But only a few are needed to keep healthy.

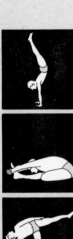

Adho Mukha Vrksasana	Goraksasana – cowherd
Ardha Baddha Padma Paschimottanasana	Hanumanasana
Ardha Chandrasana – half moon	Kapotasana – pigeon
Baddha Padmasana – bound lotus	Krounchasana – heron
Dhanurasana – bow	Kukkutasana – cock
Eka Pada Sarvangasana	Kurmasana – tortoise
Eka Pada Urdhva Dhanurasana	Marichyasana I

Matsyasana
– fish

Supta
Konasana

Natarajasana
– lord of the dance

Triang
Mukhaikapada
Paschimottanasana

Parighasana
– cross-beam

Ubhaya
Padangusthasana

Parivrtta
Parsvakonasana

Utkatasana

Parivrttaika
Pada Sirsasana

Uttana
Mayurasana
– peacock

Parsva
Halasana

Uttanasana

Purvottanasana

Uttihita Hasta
Padangusthasana

Rajakapotasana
– king of pigeons

Virabhadrasana III

Yoga for health

Yoga is such a thorough system of exercise for the whole body that regular practice of a few selected postures will help to correct and prevent almost any disorder.

People with back troubles and stiff joints will notice an improvement, since yoga works particularly on the spine, muscles and joints. Yoga relaxes tensions set up in the body by psychological causes, so can eliminate the "mysterious" headaches, stomach problems and other aches and pains which have no obvious physical basis.

Some of the common minor ailments that yoga can cure are: bad circulation, indigestion, constipation, overweight, bad posture, fatigue, sleeplessness, and menstrual pain. If you are free of these troubles, then yoga will keep you that way!

If you have a more serious complaint, such as very high blood pressure, slipped disc or heart disease, then consult your doctor and a qualified teacher before doing yoga. Yoga can help, but it is important to get expert advice on the postures that are beneficial and those which may be dangerous.

The following is a list of common problems, with a selection of postures which are particularly beneficial. Only postures illustrated in this book are listed.

Ankles, weak: the standing postures, Virasana, Baddha Konasana, Bharadvajasana, Salabhasana, Ustrasana.

Arthritis, in lower back: the standing postures, Uttanasana, Sarvangasana, Bharadvajasana, Marichyasana, Ardha Matsyendrasana, Salabhasana.

Arthritis, dorsal: the standing postures, Paschimottanasana, Bhujangasana, Adho Mukha Svanasana, Sarvangasana, Bharadvajasana, Marichyasana, Ardha Matsyendrasana.

Arthritis, shoulders: the standing postures, Halasana, Virasana, Paschimottanasana, Ardha Matsyendrasana, Bharadvajasana.

Backache: Sarvangasana, the standing postures, Jatara Parivartanasana, Janu Sirsasana, Paschimottanasana, Ardha Matsyendrasana, Ustrasana, Salabhasana.

Blood pressure (low): Sirsasana.

Blood pressure (high): Halasana, Sarvangasana, Paschimottanasana.

Constipation: Sirsasana, Sarvangasana; the standing postures, Paschimottanasana, Jatara Parivartanasana.

Fatigue: Sarvangasana, Halasana, Paschimottanasana, Uttanasana, Sirsasana, Savasana.

Headache: Sirsasana, Sarvangasana, Halasana, Paschimottanasana, Uttanasana, Savasana.

Indigestion: the standing postures, Sirsasana, Sarvangasana, Jatara Parivartanasana, Navasana, Salabhasana, Paschimottanasana, Supta Virasana.

Insomnia: Sirsasana, Sarvangasana, Paschimottanasana, Uttanasana, Savasana.

Labour (and throughout pregnancy): Virasana, Baddha Konasana, Savasana, Upavistha Konasana.

Menstrual difficulties: Sirsasana, Sarvangasana (these two not during menstruation), Paschimottanasana, Uttanasana, Virasana, Baddha Konasana, Upavistha Konasana.

Round shoulders: the standing postures, Salabhasana, Ustrasana, Padangusthasana, Uttanasana, Bhujangasana, Adho Mukha Svanasana, Janu Sirsasana, Upavistha Konasana, Bharavadjasana, Marichyasana, Ardha Matsyendrasana, Jatara Parivartanasana.

Slipped disc (but consult your doctor and a good yoga teacher): the standing postures, Padangusthasana, Paschimottanasana, Salabhasana, Ustrasana, Bhujangasana, Adho Mukha Svanasana, Sarvangasana.

Uterus, displaced: Sarvangasana, Sirsasana, Uttanasana, Padangusthasana, Dandasana, Baddha Konasana, Upavistha Konasana.

Meditation
Some of the physical effects of meditation are the slowing down of the metabolism, lowering of blood pressure and heart rate and an increase in blood flow. Meditation can be very helpful for people with high blood pressure and for those with any form of anxiety or nervous tension.
A full list of postures for therapeutic purposes can be found in B. K. S. Iyengar's book *Light on Yoga*.

Book list

CLASSICS

The yoga classics are now available in many editions and translations. The **Upanishads** and the **Bhagavadgita** are both available in the Penguin Classics series, in a very readable translation by Juan Mascaro, £0.50p each. A good paperback version of Patanjali's **Yoga Sutras** is **Aphorisms of Yoga**, commentary by Shree Purohit Swami, Faber and Faber, £0.95p.

The most famous classical commentaries on Patanjali are by Vyasa and Shankara.

The Yoga of Light, Hatha Yoga Pradipika, India's classical handbook, commentary by Hans-Ulrich Rieker, Allen & Unwin, £2.95.

GENERAL

Yoga, Ernest Wood, Penguin, £0.60.
An academic approach, with many insights, but not very concise. Best read in conjunction with a more practical book.

Textbook of Yoga, Georg Feuerstein, Rider and Company,
A broad, systematic outline of the history and development of the many forms of yoga.

Yoga, James Hewitt, Hodder and Stoughton, £0.60p.
A clear, practical introduction to yoga.

Yoga, a Way of Life, Ronald Hutchinson, Hamlyn £2.25.
A glossy, colourful book, written in a simple style, illustrating the relevance of yoga to modern living.

MEDITATION

Guide to Yoga Meditation, Richard Hittleman, Bantam Books, £0.60p.
Simple and readable, with illustrations.

Meditations from the Tantras, Swami Satyananda Saraswati, Bihar School of Yoga, £2.00.
Detailed book on meditation by the disciple of Sivananda which contains a useful introduction to the theory of meditation.

HINDUISM

Hinduism, A C Bouquet, Hutchinson University Library, £1.95. Rather a 'western' approach, but good on history.

The Hindu View of Life, Radhakrishnan, Allen & Unwin Books, £0.50p.
A short but slightly waffly book by one of India's leading modern philosophers.

HISTORY AND PHILOSOPHY

The Philosophical Traditions of India, P T Raju, Allen & Unwin, £3.95.
A clear and concise history of Indian philosophy.

Written for undergraduates, and very readable.

The Six Systems of Indian Philosophy, Max Muller, Longmans, £5.00.
One of the first modern studies of Indian philosophy (1899). A huge work, only for the keen historian, but very readable. Though scholarly, it is not at all heavy and has a pleasant period flavour.

Yoga: Immortality and Freedom, Mircea Eliade, Routledge and Kegan Paul, £7.50.
A somewhat demanding academic work, but a very comprehensive study of yoga.

For works by modern Indian philosophers, look for Aurobindo, Krishnamurti (there is a **Penguin Krishnamurti Reader**), Sivananda, Vivekenanda.

HATHA YOGA

Hatha Yoga, Theos Bernard, Rider, £1.30.

The Serpent Power, Sir John Woodroff, Ganesh, £0.60.

Light on Yoga, B K S Iyengar, Allen & Unwin, £3.50.
The most complete book on the Hatha Yoga asanas with more than six hundred illustrations. There is a section on Pranayama and an introduction to the philosophical and technical aspects of yoga. Foreword by Yehudi Menuhin.

Surya Namaskars, An Ancient Indian Exercise, Apa Pant, Orient Longmans.

Fundamentals of Yoga, Dr Rammurti Mishra, Lyrebird Press, £2.50.
One of the best contemporary books on yoga.

'COMPARATIVE' PHILOSOPHY

The Tibetan Book of the Dead, W Y Evans-Wentz, Oxford University Press, £1.75.

The Way of Zen and **Psychotherapy East and West,** Alan Watts, Penguin, both £0.40p.

Yoga and Western Psychology, Geraldine Coster, Harper Colophon.

Modern Man in Search of a Soul, Carl Jung, Routledge and Kegan Paul, £1.25.

The Perennial Philosophy, Aldous Huxley, Chatto, £2.25.

The Phenomenon of Man, Teilhard de Chardin, Fontana, £0.50p.

A Psychiatrist Discovers India, Prof. Medard Boss, Wolff, £2.25.

Lateral Thinking, Edward de Bono, Ward Lock Educational, £2.75.

Beyond Good and Evil, Friedrich Nietzsche, Penguin, £0.60p.

Supernature and **The Romeo Error,** Lyall Watson, Hodder, both £3.25.

Small is Beautiful, E F Schumacher, Abacus, £1.50.

Courses & useful addresses

There are a large number of courses available for those who wish to pursue a study of yoga. Many of these are offered as evening classes by local education authorities who should be consulted over programmes.

Listed below are the addresses of a number of individuals and organizations who will help with the many and varied applications of yoga. The list is by no means complete and the interested reader will find that contact with those involved in the subject will lead to a rapidly widening circle of connections.

The Wheel of Yoga is a co-ordinating organization mainly operating in the UK but with members in many countries overseas. Activities include public meetings, instructional seminars on all aspects of yoga, supervising of yoga teacher education, co-operation with local educational authorities in yoga tuition, and the publication of literature.

The Wheel is a registered educational trust directed by its officers and a committee representing regions in the UK with several co-opted members. It publishes The British Wheel of Yoga.
Secretary General:
Vivian Worthington,
Glyn Galleries,
Glyn Ceiriog,
Llangollen,
Clwyd.

Assistant Secretary:
Ken Thompson,
171 Chester Road,
Seven Kings,
Ilford,
Essex.

Velta Wilson,
46 Crouch Hall Road,
London N8 8HJ.

Hindu Centre,
39 Grafton Terrace,
London NW5.

Robert Hughes,
(Specializes in working with mentally ill),
Hartfield House,
50 Palace Road,
London SW2.

Centre for Transcendental Meditation,
5 Iddeslegigh House,
Caxton Street,
London SW1.

Centre House,
10a Airlie Gardens,
London W8.

Sri Chinmoy Centre,
31 Niagara Avenue,
London W5.

The Buddhist Society,
58 Eccleston Square,
London SW1.

The Yoga Studio,
6 Manchester Square,
London W1.

Sivananda Centre,
33 Albany Street,
London W1.

London Yoga Centre,
26 Northside,
London SW16.

Yoga for Health Clubs,
9 Old Bond Street,
London W1.

B.K.S. Iyengar Teachers'
Association,
c/o St Petersburg Place,
London W2.

Rajneesh Meditation Centre,
82 Bell Street,
London NW1.

Muktananda Centre,
Sri Gurudev Med Ashram,
Coxhill,
Chobham,
Surrey.

Kundalini Research
Foundation,
48 Nutley Avenue,
Saltdean,
Sussex.

Dev Murti Centre,
Highfield,
Lenham,
Nr Maidstone,
Kent.

Manchester and District
Yoga Society,
12 Cote Green Road,
Marple Bridge,
Cheshire.

Braeside Yoga Centre,
252 Strine Road,
Strines,
Cheshire.

F.R.Y.O.G.,
Friends of Yoga Society,
Wilfred Clark,
8 Poplar Drive,
Wotton Hall,
Nr Solihull,
Warwick.

Scottish Yoga Association,
Melkridge,
12 Dalkeith Street,
Edinburgh.

Scottish Yoga Centre,
106 St. Stephens Street,
Edinburgh.

Sanskrit is the ancient language of the Ayrans, the oldest known language of the Indo-European group. It means "cultured" or "aristocratic" language, and was probably a living language until the first few centuries AD. It is regarded as India's sacred language, since her scriptures are written in Sanskrit. It is closely related to ancient Iranian, and the characters come from the old Semitic alphabet.

Abhyasa : practice.
Advaita : non-dual, as applied to Vedanta philosophy which recognises only one reality.
Ahamkara : ego, sense of "I".
Ahimsa : non-violence, the first of the Yama.
Ajna Chakra : the Chakra situated between the eyebrows.
Anahata Chakra : the Chakra located in the heart region.
Ananda : bliss, ultimate reality.
Apana : one of the body's five "vital airs", operating in the pelvic region.
Arjuna : warrior and disciple of the god Krishna to whom the advice in the Bhagavadgita is offered.
Asamprajnata Samadhi : Pure consciousness (Samadhi) without reference to any object or idea.
Asana : posture or seat.
Ashram : a retreat, place for the study of yoga under a teacher.
Astanga yoga : the yoga system (described by Patanjali) consisting of eight "limbs" or overlapping interdependent stages.
Asteya : abstinence from stealing, one of the five Yama.
Astika : orthodox Hindu philosophical system.
Atman : Brahman as manifested in the individual, the self.
Aum : om, the sacred syllable representing Brahman. The supreme mantra.

Bandha : muscular contraction used in Hatha yoga, sometimes closing exits such as throat or anus.
Basti (or vasti) : one of the purification practices of Hatha yoga, for cleaning the intestines.
Bhagava : lord.
Bhagavadgita : great work on yoga of sixth century BC, part of the epic Mahabharata.
Bhakti : worship, devotion.
Bhakti yoga : yoga of devotion or worship.
Bhastrika : the "Bellows" breath, form of rapid breathing.
Bija : seed, object for meditation.
Bija Mantra : short mantra associated with one of the Chakras.
Brahma : the creative aspect of Brahman, first of the Hindu trinity of gods.
Brahma Sutras : the Sutras (concise statements) summarising the Vedanta philosophy, ascribed to Badarayana.
Brahmacharya : sexual abstinence or continence.
Brahman : the Absolute, Supreme Reality.
Brahmin : member of priestly class of Hindus.
Buddha : sixth century BC, founder of Buddhism.

Chakra : literally wheel; centre of vital energy in body.
Chela : student, disciple.
Chit : pure consciousness.
Chitta : total structure of the mind including all forms of consciousness.

Darsana : perception (of Truth), used to denote a philosophy.

Deva: a god.
Devi: a goddess.
Dharana: concentration, sixth limb of yoga.
Dhauti: one of purification practices of Hatha yoga, swallowing strip of cloth to cleanse stomach.
Dhyana: contemplation, seventh limb of yoga.
Duhkha: suffering.
Dvesha: hatred or aversion, one of the Kleshas.

Ekagra: a focused state of mind in concentration. "One-pointedness."

Gheranda Samhita: old work on Hatha yoga.
Gita: see Bhagavadgita.
Goraksanatha: supposed founder of Hatha yoga.
Goraksa Samhita: old work on Hatha Yoga.
Guna: literally rope. One of three cosmic qualities or forces which make up whole of nature.
Guru: teacher, guide, especially relating to spiritual matters.

Ha: sun.
Hatha: effort, force; sun-moon.
Hatha yoga: physical yoga.

Ida Nadi: channel or "nerve" conducting Prana from left nostril down left side of spinal cord.
Indra: warrior god of the Vedas.
Indriya: the senses.
Ishvara: God, the personal manifestation of Brahman.
Ishvarakrishna: author of commentary on Kapila's lost Sutras, setting out Samkhya philosophy.
Ishvara Pranidhana: devotion to God, one of the Niyama.

Jalandara Bandha: chinlock in Hatha yoga.
Japa: repetition of mantras.
Jiva: individual soul.
Jivanmukta: liberated soul still living in human body.
Jivatman: manifestation of Brahman in the individual soul.
Jnana: higher knowledge, especially spiritual knowledge.
Jnana Mudra: gesture of thumb and forefinger forming a circle, used in meditation.
Kala: time.
Kaivalya: liberation of soul.
Kanda: resting place of Kundalini, a short distance above the anus.
Kapila: author of original Samkhya Sutras.
Karma: action and the effects of action.
Karma yoga: the yoga of detachment from the results of one's actions.
Krishna: a divine incarnation, the speaker in the Bhagavadgita.
Kriya: action.
Kumbhaka: retention of breath.
Kundalini: vital force at base of spine, represented as coiled sleeping serpent.

Laya: absorption, falling into sleep.
Laya yoga: yoga in which bodily functions cease, releasing energy for inner experience of Samadhi.
Lingam: phallic symbol.

Mahabharata: ancient epic, of which Bhagavadgita is part.
Mahadeva: "great god", Shiva.
Mahavira: founder of Jainism.
Maithuna: ritual sexual intercourse as practised in Tantra.
Manas: the lower mind. Intellectual reasoning, selection and sense control.
Mandala: sacred symbols of universe within circle and square.
Manipura: the Chakra in the region of the solar plexus.
Mantra: sacred sound repeated in meditation.
Marga: path to spiritual goal.
Maya: in Vedanta, creative force of cosmos, sometimes translated as illusion.
Meru: in mythology the mountain supporting the world. In Hatha yoga the centre of the spinal cord.
Mimamsa: one of the six Hindu systems of philosophy.
Moksa: liberation of the soul.
Mudra: gesture or posture designed to stimulate and control psychic energy.
Mukti: liberation of soul
Muladhara: the lowest Chakra, at the base of the spine.
Muni: sage.

Nada: mystic sound of universe.
Nadi: channel in subtle body through which Prana flows.
Narayana: a name for Vishnu.
Nastika: unorthodox, referring to Buddhism and Jainism.
Nauli: one of purification practices of Hatha yoga, an abdominal exercise.
Neti: purification practice for cleansing nose.
Nirvana: enlightenment or liberation of soul, when desires cease, used especially in Buddhism.
Niyama: five observances, part of ethcial rules for all yogis. The second of the eight "limbs" of classical yoga.
Nyaya: one of the six Hindu philosophical systems.

Om: see Aum.

Padma: lotus.
Padmasana: lotus seat.
Pandit: title of learning.
Paramatma: the supreme Self.
Parinama: transformation of Prakriti world.
Pingala Nadi: channel conducting Prana from right nostril down right side of spine.
Prakriti: the most suitable form of nature, the cosmos.
Pralaya: periodic dissolution of the world.
Prana: breath, life force.
Pranavah: name of God, Om.

Pranayama : breath control.
Pratyahara : sense withdrawal.
Puraka : breathing in.
Puranas : books of ancient legends about creation of world.
Purusa : supreme consciousness or the individual soul.

Raja yoga : yoga of mind control.
Rajas : one of the three Gunas, cosmic force of motion.
Rama : A legendary Hindu king, believed to be a divine reincarnation and the hero of the epic Ramayana.
Rechaka : breathing out.
Rishi : seer. The Rishis gave voice to the Vedas, from divine inspiration.
Rudra : god, a form of Shiva.

Sahasrara Chakra : Chakra at crown of the head.
Samadhi : state of superconsciousness, last of eight limbs of yoga.
Samkhya : the Hindu system of philosophy on which the Yoga Sutras of Patanjali were developed. Samkhya means scientific knowledge.
Samprajnata Samadhi : super-consciousness achieved with the aid of an object or idea to fix the mind.
Samsara : the wheel of reincarnation.
Samskaras : impressions in the unconscious mind.
Samyama : practice of meditation, the last three limbs of yoga together: Dharana, Dhyana and Samadhi.
Santosha : contentment, one of the five Niyamas.
Sat : reality, truth.
Sattva : one of the three Gunas, cosmic force of consciousness and order.
Satya : truthfulness, one of the five Yama.
Shakti : creative power; goddess representing this power.
Shanti : peace.

Shivasamhita : book on Hatha yoga.
Shri : polite form of address.
Shunyaka : holding an exhalation.
Siddha : "perfected one", possessor of occult powers.
Siddhi : power (esp. occult).
Siddhasana : perfect posture, used for meditation.
Sirsasana : headstand.
Sharira : body. There are three bodies: dense, subtle and causal.
Shastra : scripture.
Shatkarma : six purification practices of Hatha yoga.
Shiva : third god in Hindu trinity, the Transformer of life.
Sruti : scriptures, divine revelations, such as Vedas.
Surya Namaskars : Salute to the Sun, a Hatha yoga exercise.
Susumma : most important of the Nadis, and path of Kundalini, through centre of spinal column and main Chakras.
Sutras : condensed statements summarizing a philosophy.
Swadhyaya : study, esp. self-knowledge, one of the five Niyama.
Swadisthana : the Chakra near the reproductive organs.
Swami : renunciate.
Swatmarama : author of Hatha Yoga Pradipika.

Tad Ekam : "that one", refers to Brahman.
Tamas : cosmic force of darkness and inertia. One of the three Gunas.
Tanmatras : units of energy prior to creation of sensible phenomena.
Tantras : scriptures on religious ritual worship and meditation.
Tapas : discipline, esp. of body.
Tat : that, Brahman.
Tattva : thatness; the truth about something; also an element evolved from the Gunas.
Tattvam : reality, oneness.
Tat Tvam Asi : That Thou Art, statement from the Upanishads

expressing identity of God and individual soul.
Tha : moon.
Trataka : steady gaze at an object for eye exercise or meditation.
Udana : one of five "vital airs" in the body.
Ujjayi : a technique of controlled audible breathing.
Upanishads : latest part of Vedas, source of Vedanta philosophy.

Vairagya : "uncolouredness." Dispassionate condition of mind.
Vaisesika : one of six Hindu philosophical systems.
Vasistha : see Yoga Vasistha.
Vedas : ancient Indian literature, collection of hymns and scriptures. There are four Vedas: Rig Veda, Yajur Veda, Sama Veda, Atharva Veda.
Vedanta : Hindu philosophy which is most widely held. The ultimate form of the Vedas.
Vishnu : second god in Hindu trinity, the Preserver of life.
Visuddha : Chakra at the throat.
Viveka : Samkhya term: discrimination between ego and Self.
Vratyas : ancient brotherhood mentioned in Vedas, possibly early yogis.
Vritti : modifications of activity of the mind.

Yama : five rules of conduct forming, with Niyama, basic ethical code for yogis.
Yantra : a visual aid to meditation constructed from a geometric pattern of triangles within a circle within a square.
Yogarudha : "mounted on yoga", practised yogi.
Yoga Upanishads : post-classical work on yoga.
Yoga Vasistha : philosophical work on yoga by Valmiki.
Yogi, Yogin : one who practises yoga.
Yogini : female yogi.

Index

Numbers in italics indicate
illustrations

Abhyasa, 13, 22
Absolute, the, 7
Ahimsa, 9
Arjuna, 7, *9*, 14, 30
Aryan tribes, 6
Asanas, 18, 21, 22, 33, 34
  Adho Mukha Svanasana,
  54, 84, 85
  84, 85
  Anantasana, 77, 85
  ArdhaMatsyendrasana I,
  72, 85
  Ardha Padmasana, 79
  Baddha Konasana, 49,
  84, 85
  Bharadvajasana I, 52, 70,
  84, 85
  Bhujangasana, 53, 84, 85
  Chakrasana, 76
  Dandasana, 45, 84, 85
  Halasana, 60, 84
  Janu Sirsasana, 48, 84,
  85
  Jathara Parivartanasana,
  56, 84, 85
  Karnapidasana, 62
  Marichyasana III, 70, 85
  Matsyasana, 87
  Natarajasana, 87
  Padangusthasana, 67, 85
  Padmasana, 79
  Parighasana, 87
  Paripurna Navasana, 71,
  85
  Parivrttaika
  Pada Sirasasana, 87
  Parivrtta Trikonasana, 66,
  85

Parsva Halasana, 87
Parsvakonasana, 87
Parsvottanasana, 42-3, *42-3*,
84, 85
Paschimottanasana, 46, 48,
60, 84, 85
Prasarita Padottanasana, 69,
85
Purvottanasana, 87
Rajakapotasana, 87
Salabhasana, 75, 85
Salamba Sarvangasana,
58, 84
Savasana, 34, 63
Sirsasana, 78
Supta Konasana, 87
Supta Virasana, 50, 85
Surya Namaskars, 64
Tadasana, 35, 36, 84, 85
Triang Mukhaikapada
Paschimottanasana, 87
Ubhaya
Padangusthasana, 87
Upavistha Konasana, 68,
85
Urdhva Dhanurasana, 76,
85
Ustrasana, 74, 85
Utkatasana, 87
Uttana Mayurasana, 87
Uttanasana, 40, 84, 85,
87
Uttihita Hasta
Padangusthasana, 87
Uttihita Parsvakonasana,
37, 84, 85
Uttihita Trikonasana, 36,
84, 85
Virabhadrasana I, 38, 84,
85
Virabhadrasana II, 39,
84, 85
Virabhadrasana III, 87
Virasana, 50, 84, 85
Vrksasana, 41, 84, 85
Atman, 13, 34
Avidya, 10, 13, 22
Aviveka, 10

Bhagavadgita, 4, 7, 8, 14,
16, 28
Biofeedback, 26
Boat pose, 71, 85
Bound lotus pose, 86
Bow pose, 86
Brahman, 4, 7, 8, 13, 16,
20, 81

Brahmin, *22*
Breathing, 34
Brihadaranyka Upanishad,
34
Buddha, 9, *9*, *12*
Buddhism, 8, 81

Camel pose, 74, 85
Chakras, 19, 20, *20*, 25
Christ, 16
Cleansing, 18 ·
Cobbler pose, 49, 84
Cobra pose, 53, 84, 85
Cock pose, 86
Consciousness, 21
Corpse pose, 34, 63, 84
Cosmic energy, 20
Cowherd pose, 86
Cross-beam, 87

Dalai Lama, 7
Darsana, 10
Dharana, 23, 81
Dhyana, 23, 81
Dog pose, 54, 84, 85
Donne, John, 4

Electroencephalograph, 27
Elements, 20
Eternity, 15

Fakir, *23*
Fish pose, 87
Forward bend, 46, 84, 85

Gandhi, *14*
Goraksanatha, 18
Gunas, 12, 24

Ha, 21
Half moon pose, 86
Hatha Yoga Pradipika, 18,
21, 79
Headstand, 78
Hero, 84
Heron pose, 86
Hindu, 4, 6, 10
Hindu philosophy, 7, 24
Hinduism, 6, 8, 17

Ida, 19, 20, 21
Indian philosophy, 10
Indus Valley, 6
Infinity, 15
Ishvara, 22
Islam, 17

Iyengar, B.K.S., 25, 34, 71

Jain, monks, *8*
   painting, *24*
Jainism, 8, 9
Jung, 27

Kaivalya, 10
Karma, 11
Katha, Upanishad, 7
King of pigeons, 87
Krishna, *5*, 7, 8, *9*, 11, 15,
   16, *16*, 30

Locust pose, 75, 83, 85
Lord of the dance, 87
Lotus flower, *13*, 20
Lotus pose, 79, 85

Mahabharata, 7
Maharishi Mahesh Yogi, *29*
Maithuna, 17, 19
Mandala, 17
   Tibetan, *17*
Mantras, 17, 29, 82
   seed, 25
Maya, 13
Mimamsa, 10
Meditation, 22, 28, 81
Mohenjo-Daro, 6
Mountain pose, 84, 85
Mudra, 17
Mukti, 10

Nirvana, 10
Niyama, 14, 19, 22
Nyaya, 10

Occult powers, 23
Om, *23*

Patanjali, 8, 12, 13, 22, 30
Path Supreme, the, 7
Peacock pose, 87
Piezo-electricity, 27
Pingala, 19, 20, 21
Pigeon pose, 86
Plough pose, 60, 84
Postures, see Asanas
Pradipika, 20
Prakriti, 12
Pralayas, 12
Prana, 18, 19
Pranayama, 22, 80
Pratyahara, 23
Prayer wheels, *25*

Psychoanalysis, 27
Purusa, 12, 13

Qualities, 24

Rajas, 12
Ramakrishna, 7
Relaxed pose, 40, 84, 85
Religion, 4
Respiration, 33
Reverse triangle, 66, 85
Rishis, 7
Rudra, 9

Saivism, 11
Salute to the sun, 64
Samadhi, 4, 10, 14, 18, 20,
   23, 24, 25, 81
Samkhya, 10, 22, 26
Samsara, 11
Samyama, 23
Sanskrit, 4
Saraswati, Swami
   Satyananda, 28
Sattva, 12
Self, 12, 13, 24
Shakti, 17, 20, 21
Shiva, 6, 9, *11*, 17, 20, 21
Shoulder exercise, 44
Shoulder stand, 58, 84, 85
Siddha, 23
Sirsasana, 21
Spine, 20, 34, 35
Staff pose, 45, 84, 85
Subtle body, 19
Superconsciousness, 4
Susumma, 19, 20, 21

Tad Ekam, 7
Tamas, 12
Tantras, 9
Tantrism, 17
Tatt vam Asi, 7
Tha, 21
That One, 7
Toe catch, 67, 85
Tortoise, 86
Transcendental Meditation,
   29
Trataka, 17
Tree pose, 41, 84, 85
Triangle pose, 36, 84, 85
Twine pose, 52, 84

Udana, 23
Upanishads, 7, 10, 13

Vairagya, 13, 22
Vaisesika, 10
Vaisnavism, 11
Vedanta, 10, 13, 17, 81
Vedas, 6, 7, 8, 10, 13, 18
Virabhadra, 38
Vishnu, *11*
Vivekenanda, 8
Vratyas, 9

Warrior pose, 84
Wheel pose, 76, 85
Wood, Ernest, 28

Yama, 14, 19, 22
Yantra, 17
Yoga, 10
   and physics, 26
   and psychology, 27
   and science, 26
   Astanga, 22
   Bhakti, 14, 16
   class, *29*
   classical, 8, 24
   Hatha, 9, 17, 18, 20, 24
   history, 6
   in the West, 24
   Jnana, 14, 15
   Karma, 14, 15, 28
   kundalini, 20, 24
   Laya, 20
   limbs, 22, 23
   Mantra, 25
   origins, 6
   paths, 14
   philosophy, 10
   physiology, 27
   Raja, 22, 24
   Samkhya, 10, 12
   Sutras, 8, 12, 22, 81
   Tantric, 17, 19
   today, 28
   types, 14

Credits

Artists
Anne Isseyegh
QED

Models
Sophy Hoare
Syd Hoare

Photographs
Heather Angel: 13
Archiv für Kunst und
geschichte: 5, 17, 81

Chester Beatty Library: 21
John Cutten: 27
Werner Forman: 9, 24
Paul Forrester, entire
activities section
Hamlyn/Ben Rose
Photography Inc./
Scientific American
Magazine: 26
Hamlyn/Gulbenkien;
contents, 20
Hamlyn/Victoria & Albert
Museum: contents, 82
Michael Holford: contents, 11
(right), 12
Victor Kennet: 11 (left), 18
Keystone: 29
Bury Peerless: 6, 9, 11

Peter Myers: 83
Popperfoto: 7, 14, 29, 30
Camera Press: 28
Radio Times Hulton Picture
Library: 22, 23
Rhamakrishna
Vivekenanda Centre: 7, 8
(top)
Richard & Sally Greenhill: 8
(bottom)
SEF: 10, 25
Victoria & Albert Museum: 16

Cover
Design: Barry Kemp
Photograph: Margaret
Murray